Pocket Workouts

2015

N. Rey | darebee.com

Printed in the United Kingdom.

First Printing, 2015

ISBN 13: 978-1-84481-001-7

ISBN 10: 1-84481-001-1

Warning and Disclaimer

Although every precaution has been taken to verify the accuracy of
the information contained herein, the author and publisher assume no
responsibility for any errors or omissions. No liability is assumed for
damages that may result from the use of information contained within.

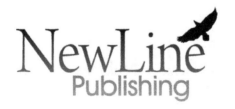

Thank you!

Thank you for purchasing *Pocket Workouts*, DAREBEE project print edition. DAREBEE is a non-profit global fitness resource dedicated to making fitness accessible for everyone, no matter the circumstances. The project is supported exclusively via user donations and paperback royalties.

After printing cost and store fees every book developed by DAREBEE project makes $1 and it goes directly into our project maintenance and development fund.

Each sale helps us keep the DAREBEE resource growing, maintain it and keep it up. Thank you for making a difference in its future!

100 workouts

1. Abs of Steel
2. Abs Unlocked
3. Abs Upgrade
4. Armor Abs
5. Code of Abs
6. Express Abs
7. Five Minute Plank
8. Good Morning, Abs
9. Ironclad Abs
10. Power Abs
11. Supernova
12. Bacon
13. That Escalated!
14. Cardio & Core
15. Cardio Hop
16. Cardio Light
17. Cardio Rock
18. Chase
19. Chisel
20. Contender
21. Dash
22. DNA:Rewrite
23. Extractor
24. Forge
25. Heist
26. Hell Raider
27. Jacks
28. Power Burpee
29. Quick Silver
30. Rebel
31. Reboot
32. Roaster
33. Scout
34. Skier
35. Spy

36. Torch
37. Ultimate Burn
38. Aim to Misbehave
39. Armageddon
40. Arms of Steel
41. Bodyguard
42. Body Hack
43. Bootcamp
44. Boss Fight
45. Boulder
46. Bounty Hunter
47. Boxer
48. Centurion
49. Combat Strength
50. Commando
51. Crucible
52. Dragon Slayer
53. Equalizer
54. Fremen
55. Gambit
56. Gladiator
57. Golem
58. Gravity
59. Guardian
60. Hercules
61. Homemade Back
62. Huntsman
63. Leg Day
64. Legs of Steel
65. Odin
66. Paladin
67. Plan B
68. Power Flow
69. Power Mode
70. Primal

71. Push, Squat, Repeat
72. Reaper
73. Reclaimer
74. Savage
75. Sculptor
76. Spartan
77. Super Soldier
78. Titan
79. Viking
80. Anchor'd
81. Balance & Coordination
82. Bowman
83. Far Point
84. Inner Warrior
85. Liber8
86. Origami
87. Stakeout
88. Express
89. Coffee Break
90. Gamer
91. Hand
92. Movie Night
93. Office
94. Sofa Abs
95. Star Master
96. Wake Up!
97. Knee
98. Lower Back
99. Man Down
100. Neck

Introduction

Bodyweight training may look easy, but if you are not used to it, it's very far from that. It is just as intense as running and it is just as challenging so if you struggle with it at the very beginning, it's perfectly ok – you will get better at it once you start doing it regularly. Do it at your own pace and take longer breaks if you need to.

You can start with a single individual workout from the collection and see how you feel. If you are new to bodyweight training always start any workout on Level I (level of difficulty).

You can pick any number of workouts per week, usually between 3 and 5 and rotate them for maximum results.

Some workouts are more suitable for weight loss and toning up and others are more strength oriented, some do both. To make it easier for you to choose, they have all been labelled according to FOCUS, use it to design a training regimen based on your goal.

High Burn and Strength oriented workouts will help you with your weight, aerobic capacity and muscle tone, some are just more specialized, but it doesn't mean you should exclusively focus on one or the other. Whatever your goal with bodyweight training you'll benefit from doing exercises that produce results in both areas.

This collection has been designed to be completely no-equipment for maximum accessibility so several bodyweight exercises like pull-ups have been excluded. If you want to work on your biceps and back more and you do have access to a pull-up bar, have one at home or can use it somewhere else like the nearest playground (monkey bars), you can do wide and close grip pull-ups, 3 sets to failure 2-3 times a week with up to 2 minutes rest in between sets in addition to your training. Alternatively, you can add pull-ups in the be
ginning or at the end of every set of a Strength Oriented workout.

All of the routines in this collection are suitable for both men and women, no age restrictions apply.

Design your training regimen

Goal: Slim down and tone up

Select workouts for "high burn" – these are the workouts you are looking for.

If you want to slim down, putting some extra muscle on will help you burn more, naturally (muscles are very high maintenance and will burn extra calories with every move you make) so strength workouts shouldn't be completely ignored.

It's worth mentioning that women won't be able to bulk up, not naturally and not without any supplements, due to the much lower levels of testosterone present in the female body. The best we can hope for is nice muscle tone and a tight... well, stuff and everything.

Important: Without dietary adjustments you will get fitter, but you won't lose body fat %, unfortunately. You can't out train a bad diet – you can't train and eat junk and hope that it will cancel out, you would have to train on athlete level and very few people can do that. If you are not running 10K daily and doing another bodyweight session after that, you will have to mind what you eat if your goal is to slim down.

Also very important: you can lose weight when you are on a diet and see it on the scales, you gain muscle as well as lose body fat % when you diet and exercise. If you work out, don't use the scales, unless they have BF% meter in them, to measure your progress. Take pictures of yourself either daily or once every few days to track how you are doing and if you need to change anything like training more or eating less, yes. Alternatively, judge by your clothes – if you need new clothes, you are doing well.

Goal: Build muscle and tone up

Select workouts for "strength" – these are the workouts you are looking for.

If you want to build up muscle, you want to do more of strength training but an occasional high burn on HIIT workout will help you reduce your body fat % even further and let you see better muscle definition.

To gain weight, especially if you are skinny, as well as exercise (options above) you will need to eat a lot more than you do now, eat regularly (every 2-3 hrs) and eat quality food. Just eating a lot in general won't do it – your body can't get anything useful out of junk food, sweets, pizza and beer. In order to build muscle, you need muscle building material – high protein rich food and complex carbohydrates.

Make sure your diet is based around real food, e.g., chicken breasts, turkey, fish, pork loin, steak, eggs, milk, cheese (in moderation), low fat plain yogurts, cottage cheese, sweet potatoes, oats and oatmeal, quinoa, spinach (all leafy greens), broccoli, kale, cauliflower, mushrooms, apples, pears, oranges, berries, tomatoes, cucumbers, peppers, rice, pasta, beans and lentils, olive oil, seeds, nuts and nut butters.

Goal: Build abs and strengthen midsection

Your midsection and your hard core abs, if you are looking for those, depend on your overall body fat percentage. Where your body will be emptying those fat cells is down to your disposition and body type but it often starts from the top down.

You have two options to get rid of the belly: starve your body for resources to force it to dig into the reserves (it'll do it after it's out of other options) or do high burn cardio workouts, HIIT workouts are best — these are also known as belly torches. You want to do both for better and faster results.

Select workouts for "abs" or "high burn" — these are the workouts you are looking for.

You can still do ab work to strengthen the muscles. The more muscles you have underneath your belly, the more you'll burn during your cardio workouts. Muscles, in general are pretty high maintenance energy (calories) wise. Just doing crunches won't do anything (at least on the surface) for you and there's no study anywhere that's shown a correlation between training a particular body part or body area and a reduction in the fat stored there.

The same exact ab work will eventually force your body into optimising and you'll see less and less of an improvement with each session unless you change things up and/or increase the numbers. So it's always a good idea to do different ab work to keep your muscles challenged and the moment you begin to find one ab exercise easy, increase the load or intensity to make it more effective. If you are breezing through your ab workout you can be sure it's not working: if you think about it, why do our bodies change? Because they have to, to make it easier for us to live.

To make any ab exercise harder, you can either add weights (do sit-ups or sitting twists with dumbbells) or just do it slower, a lot slower. Going from easier exercises like crunches to more advanced ones like moving planks, for example, will also work.

Modifications / Exercise Alternatives

If you are recovering from an injury, have a mild disability that prevents you from doing certain moves, have bad knees or are suffering from back pain and you want to avoid high impact exercises but you still want to stay active and try some of the workouts from this book, try these modifications.

The modifications will also be suitable if you are trying to keep the noise you make to a minimum – it's handy if you live in an apartment and your neighbours are ... not very understanding people.

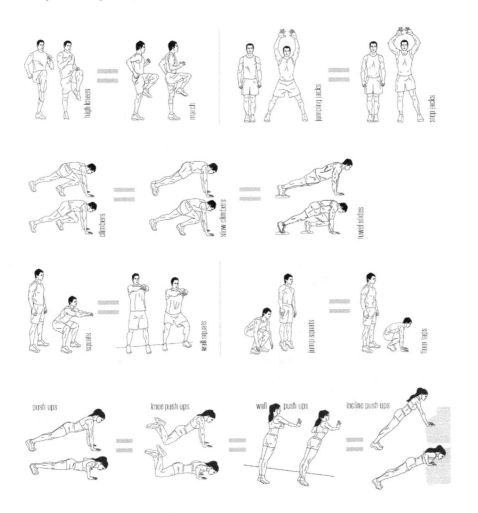

high knees — march

jumping jacks — step jacks

climbers — slow climbers — towel slides

squats — wall squats

jump squats — floor taps

push-ups — knee push-ups — wall push-ups — incline push-ups

SAMPLE WORKOUT

LEVEL I 3 sets LEVEL II 5 sets LEVEL III 7 sets REST up to 2 minutes

10 jumping jacks   **20** high knes   **40** side-to-side chops

10 squats   **20** lunges   **10-count** plank

20 climbers   **10** plank jump-ins   **to failure** push-ups

Difficulty Levels:
Level I: normal
Level II: hard
Level III: freaking murder

1 SET

10 jumping jacks
20 high knees (10 each leg)
40 side-to-side chops
(20 each side)
10 squats
20 lunges (10 each leg)
10-count plank (hold while
counting to 10)
20 climbers (10 each leg)
10 plank jump-ins
to failure push-ups
(your maximum)

**Up to 2 minutes rest
between sets:**
30 seconds,
60 seconds
or 2 minutes -
it's up to you.

Important: don't go from zero to hero. Do what you can but don't push yourself too hard too fast, just because you can do something on a harder level doesn't mean that you should. On level I all push-ups can be done on your knees.

Before you start: Look over the workout you chose to do and make sure you understand all of the exercises illustrated so it doesn't slow you down once you have started.

**Video Exercise Library
http://darebee.com/exercises**

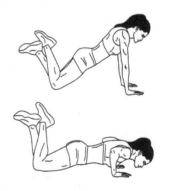

warmup

DAREBEE WORKOUT © darebee.com

10 reps each

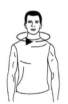
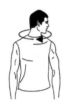

neck rotations

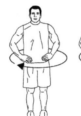
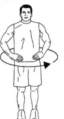

hip rotations

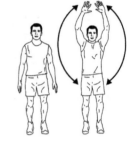

side arm raises

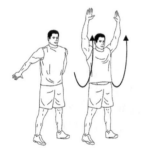

arm rotations

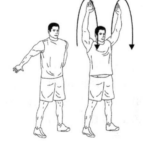

arm rotations

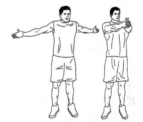

dynamic chest

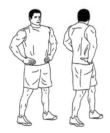

mid back turns

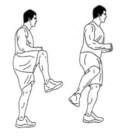

single leg hip rotations

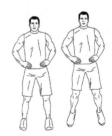

hops on the spot

1 Abs of Steel Workout

Abdominal muscles are body armour. They help protect your vital organs from damage. They keep your body performing at maximum and, when the clothes come off, they make you look terrific. This workout is the anvil where that armour is fashioned.

Tip: Always exhale when you perform any exercise that tenses the abs. This flattens your lower stomach and brings the abdominal muscles into proper alignment, increasing the pull exerted on them which strengthens them faster.

abs of steel

DAREBEE WORKOUT © darebee.com

LEVEL I 3 sets **LEVEL II** 4 sets **LEVEL III** 5 sets **REST** up to 2 minutes

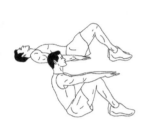

10 sit-ups

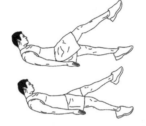

12 flutter kicks

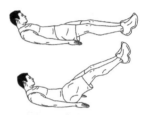

10 leg raises

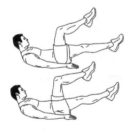

10 air bike crunches

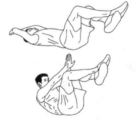

10 knee crunches

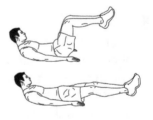

10 leg pull-ins

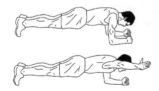

10 plank arm raises

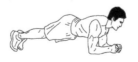

30sec elbow plank

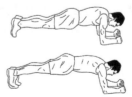

10 body saw

2   Abs Unlocked Workout

There are four major muscle groups that constitute the abdominal muscle wall and each of them does something very specific. In no particular order they are Rectus Abdominis (the frontal abs which can also be divided into upper and lower abs and make up the six-pack), External Abdominal Obliques, Internal Abdominal Obliques and Transverse Abdominis which we most popularly refer to as core. The Abs Unlocked workout works them all.

Make it harder: Reduce the rest time between sets to 90 seconds and challenge your body's ability to recover.

abs unlocked

DAREBEE WORKOUT © darebee.com

LEVEL I 3 sets **LEVEL II** 5 sets **LEVEL III** 7 sets **REST** up to 2 minutes

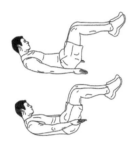

20 hundreds

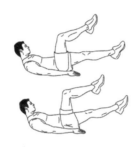

20 air bike crunches

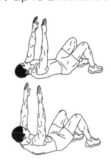

20 high crunches

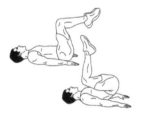

10 reverse crunches

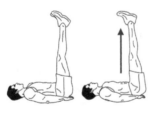

10 pulse-ups

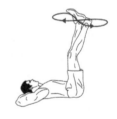

10 infinity circles

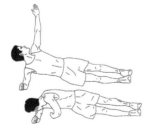

10 side plank rotations

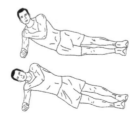

10 side bridges

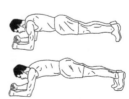

10 body saw

3   Abs Upgrade Workout

Abs are not just the engine that powers some of your most energetic movements, they also play a vital role in protecting a vulnerable part of your body. The Abs Upgrade workout works each of the four major abdominal muscle groups for that all-in feeling.

Make it better: Add some light ankle weights to this for an improved feeling.

abs upgrade

DAREBEE WORKOUT © darebee.com

LEVEL I 3 sets **LEVEL II** 4 sets **LEVEL III** 5 sets **REST** up to 2 minutes

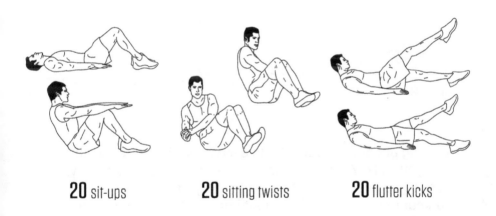

20 sit-ups **20** sitting twists **20** flutter kicks

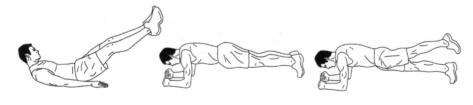

20-count raised leg hold **20-count** plank **20-count** raised leg plank

4   Armor Abs Workout

A strong abdominal wall affects everything. The way you sit. How you walk. Your performance in every kind of sport. How quickly you get tired and how smoothly you move. This is a workout that presses all the right buttons, helping you tone up and build your abs, plus come summer you're going to be thankful you did it.

Tip: The secret to better abs, faster lies in alignment. If you can remember to pull in and tighten your lower abs every time you perform an ab exercise you will see great results, faster.

armor abs

DAREBEE WORKOUT © darebee.com

LEVEL I 3 sets **LEVEL II** 5 sets **LEVEL III** 7 sets **REST** up to 2 minutes

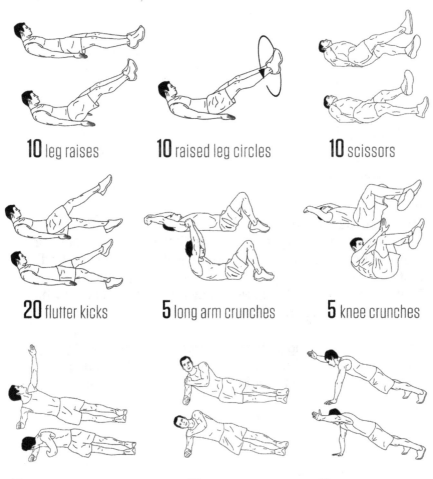

10 leg raises   **10** raised leg circles   **10** scissors

20 flutter kicks   **5** long arm crunches   **5** knee crunches

10 side planks rotations   **10** side bridges   **10** plank arm raises

5   Code of Abs Workout

The code, the source code. Strong abs are not just the engine that powers your every move nor are they just the armour that protects some of your vital organs. They're also the scaffolding that supports your spine. In short they're really important. That's why you need them. Plus they make you look cool when you take your shirt off.

Tip: When performing each of the exercises here consciously tighten your lower abs, flattening your stomach and aligning the abdominal muscle wall, for better results.

code of **abs**

DAREBEE WORKOUT © darebee.com

LEVEL I 3 sets **LEVEL II** 4 sets **LEVEL III** 5 sets **REST** up to 2 minutes

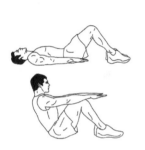

10 sit-ups

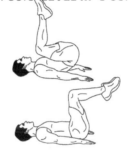

10 reverse crunches

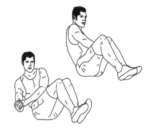

10 sitting twists

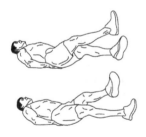

8 scissors

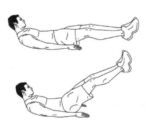

8 leg raises

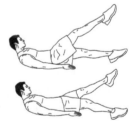

20 flutter kicks

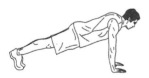

30sec plank

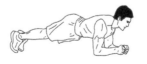

30sec elbow plank

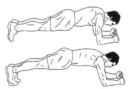

8 body saw

6   Express Abs Workout

There are four main muscle groups that make up the ab wall in its totality and Abs Express is designed to help you test each one of them for better, faster results. When it comes to building quality abs there really is no shortcut. This set of exercises will help you get there, all you have to do is put in the time and do the work.

Make it harder: Add some light ankle weights and feel your abs burn just a little bit more.

express abs

REPEAT ONCE | DAREBEE WORKOUT © darebee.com

LEVEL I 6 reps **LEVEL II** 10 reps each **LEVEL III** 20 reps each
LEVEL I 6-count hold **LEVEL II** 10-count hold **LEVEL III** 20-count hold

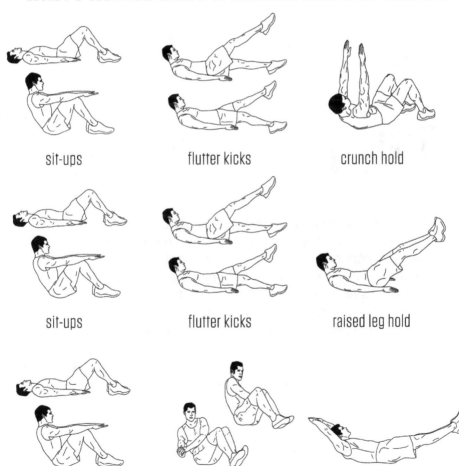

sit-ups	flutter kicks	crunch hold
sit-ups	flutter kicks	raised leg hold
sit-ups	sitting twists	hollow hold

7   Five Minute Plank Workout

Training the abdominal muscle group is no easy task. The muscles do not all respond to training at the same rate and there is a core group of abdominal s, running beneath the external ones with muscle fibres pointing the opposite way. This makes for a core picture which no single exercise can adequately address which helps explain why strong abs are hard to attain, which makes them an aim to strive for.

Tip: To gain the maximum out of your time in this exercise tense your abdominal muscle group at each rep.

FIVE MINUTE PLANK

DAREBEE WORKOUT © darebee.com

LEVEL I 3 sets **LEVEL II** 5 sets **LEVEL III** 7 sets **REST** up to 2 minutes

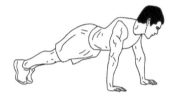

60sec full plank

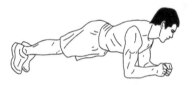

30sec elbow plank

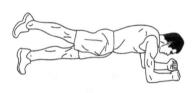

60sec raised leg plank
30 seconds - each leg

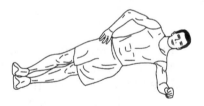

60sec side plank
30 seconds - each side

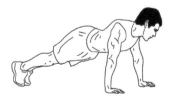

30sec full plank

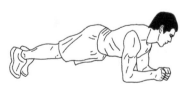

60sec elbow plank

8 Good Morning, Abs Workout

Abs are core to any kind of workout and this Morning abs routine can be performed first thing int he day before you get out of bed or last thing at night before you close your eyes and unplug from the conscious world. Ok, you can't be cozily tucked in under the blankets and do it, but you've worked that bit out already.

Make it harder: Do it twice in the day, both morning and night.

Good morning, abs

DAREBEE WORKOUT © darebee.com

LEVEL I 3 sets **LEVEL II** 4 sets **LEVEL III** 5 sets **REST** up to 2 minutes

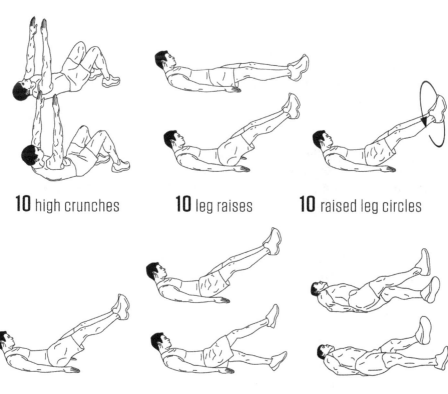

10 high crunches   **10** leg raises   **10** raised leg circles

10-count raised leg hold   **10** flutter kicks   **10** scissors

9   Ironclad Abs Workout

What you really want to do with your abs is transform them into a wall of protective, empowering muscle. There is no real shortcut you can take here. You need to do the work and feel the results. The Ironclad abs workout is perfect for giving you the results you need.

Make it better: Keep your head off the floor and your chin on your chest for every exercise where you lie on your back.

ironclad abs

DAREBEE WORKOUT © darebee.com

LEVEL I 3 sets **LEVEL II** 4 sets **LEVEL III** 5 sets **REST** up to 2 minutes

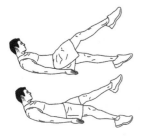

10 flutter kicks

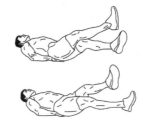

4 scissors

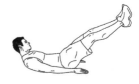

10-count hold

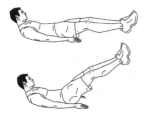

10 leg raises

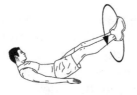

4 raised leg circles

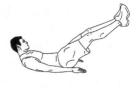

10-count hold

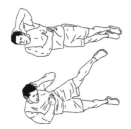

10 jackknives

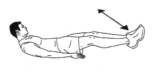

4 raised leg swings

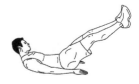

10-count hold

10   Power Abs Workout

The abdominal muscle wall is made up of four, distinct muscle groups: obliques (interior and exterior), front abdominals (rectus abdominis), and core abdominals (transverse abdominis). The Power Abs workout uses exercises that activate all of those muscle groups helping your body develop a powerful abdominal wall that will take your physical ability to an entirely new level. Perfect for those looking for an abs workout that will use every ab wall muscle group, it is also useful for leveling up on physical performance by unlocking the body's full potential.

power abs

DAREBEE WORKOUT © darebee.com

LEVEL I 3 sets **LEVEL II** 4 sets **LEVEL III** 5 sets **REST** up to 2 minutes

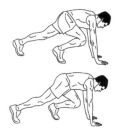

20 climbers

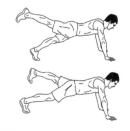

20 plank leg raises

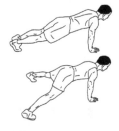

20 plank jacks

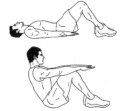

10 sit-ups

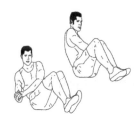

10 sitting twists

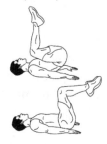

10 reverse crunches

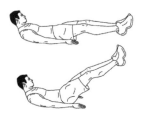

10 leg raises

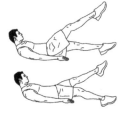

10 fluter kicks

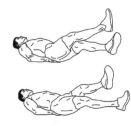

10 scissors

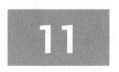 Supernova Workout

Supernovas are super-bright stars in the celestial horizon, burning high with energy being released, and this workout is designed to make you one on Earth with the kind of six-pack that'll get you noticed.

Tip: A moving plank challenges your core and helps you develop greater stability. Make sure your abs are tense throughout the movement.

super**nova**

DAREBEE WORKOUT © darebee.com

ABS & CORE

LEVEL I 3 sets **LEVEL II** 5 sets **LEVEL III** 7 sets **REST** up to 2 minutes

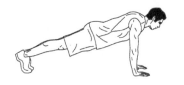

MOVE 1
20 second plank

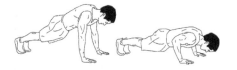

MOVE 2
10 alt arm/leg planks

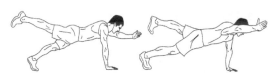

MOVE 3
4 moving plank 90 °

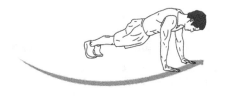

MOVE 4
20 climbers

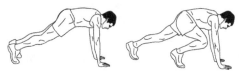

MOVE 5
10 push-ups

12   Bacon Workout

Also known as "The Belly Burner" workout this is designed to make you lean and mean. You will work up a sweat doing it. Your body will feel numb, your lungs will feel on fire and you will feel like you're being put through your paces. But ... you know it's worth it, and you're doing it for bacon. How cool is that?

Tip: You can take the entire set up a notch and do your legs a favour by making sure your heels never touch the floor on any of the exercises. That means doing everything on the balls of your feet, at all times. Your legs will love you for it later. ...Much Later.

YOU HAD ME AT
bacon

DAREBEE WORKOUT © darebee.com

LEVEL I 3 sets **LEVEL II** 5 sets **LEVEL III** 7 sets **REST** up to 2 minutes

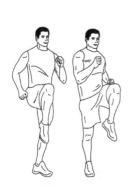

20 high knees

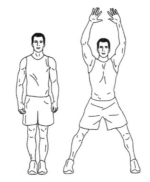

20 jumping jacks

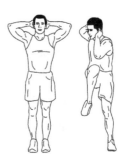

20 knee-to-elbows

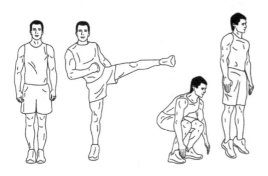

40 side leg raises

10 jump squats

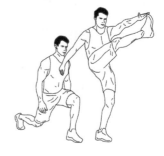

10 reverse lunge kicks

13   That Escalated! Workout

There are days when all you want to do is empty your mind and then 'empty' your body into an activity that simply works you physically until you're done. Well, look no further than this workout for that. It may not appear very challenging at first glance but you will find that it presses all the right buttons.

Make it better: Speed up the jumping jacks, pulling your arms down to your sides, instead of letting them drop down, and then work your muscles to stop them from slapping against your thighs, increasing the effectiveness of the workout on your upper body.

BOY, THAT ESCALATED QUICKLY

DAREBEE WORKOUT
© darebee.com

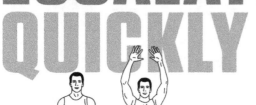

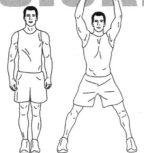

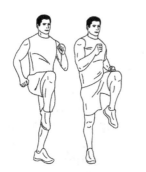

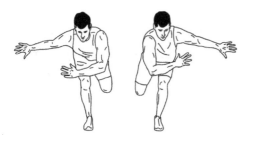

10 jumping jacks

10 high knees

10 side-to-side jumps

20 jumping jacks

20 high knees

20 side-to-side jumps

30 jumping jacks

30 high knees

30 side-to-side jumps

done

LEVEL I 3 sets
LEVEL II 5 sets
LEVEL III 7 sets
REST up to 2 minutes

14   Cardio & Core Workout

At the core of every great athletic performance lies a strong core (pun unintended) and great cardiovascular conditioning. While aerobic performance determines just how much oxygen in each breath you take is really absorbed by the lungs and transferred into the bloodstream to be taken to the organs that need it, cardiovascular fitness is the ability of the heart and lungs to get all the blood circulating quickly enough through the body to supply oxygen to the organs and tissues that need it most.

Make it better: When performing High Knees bring your knees to waist height for that very special burn on your calves and lungs.

Cardio & Core

DAREBEE WORKOUT © darebee.com

LEVEL I 3 sets **LEVEL II** 5 sets **LEVEL III** 7 sets **REST** up to 2 minutes

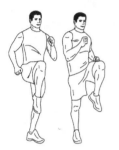

60 high knees

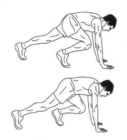

10 climbers

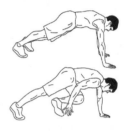

10 climber taps

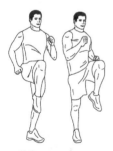

60 high knees

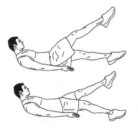

10 flutter kicks

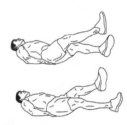

10 scissors

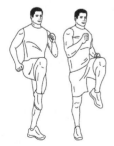

60 high knees

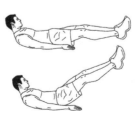

10 leg raises

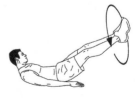

10 raised leg circles

15 Cardio Hop Workout

A cardio-burn workout doesn't necessarily have to hit insanity levels to work. As a matter of fact one that doesn't and still gets your body moving and your circulation going is ideally suited for doing as often as possible. The Cardio Hop workout is specifically designed in coordination with the NHS (British National Health service) specialists to deliver a workout that can be done any place anywhere to get your heart rate up. All you need is a little space and just a little bit of time and you're good to go.

Cardio Hop

DAREBEE WORKOUT © darebee.com
Repeat 3 times | up to 2min rest between sets

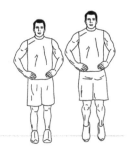

10 hop on the spot

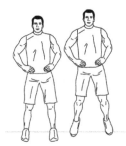

10 wide leg hops

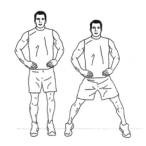

10 half jack hops

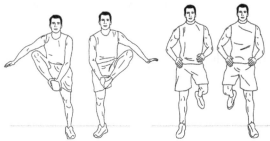

10 toe tap hops

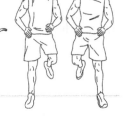

10 side-to-side single leg jumps

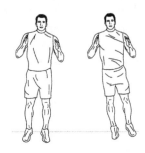

10 side-to-side hops

16   Cardio Light Workout

There are times when you want to workout and barely have the energy to get going. For those times the Cardio Light, will get you buzzing in just the right way. Designed to get your body going and your heart thumping without pushing you too hard, this is just the kind of go-to workout you go to, when you're low and really need a pick-me-up.

Make it better: Move arms and legs in unison when marching.

Cardio light

DAREBEE WORKOUT © darebee.com

LEVEL I 3 sets **LEVEL II** 5 sets **LEVEL III** 7 sets **REST** up to 2 minutes

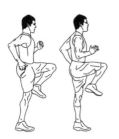

10 march steps

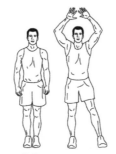

20 step jacks

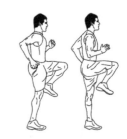

10 march steps

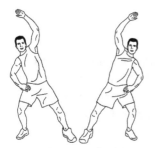

20 side jacks

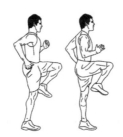

10 march steps

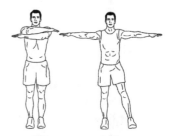

20 scissor steps

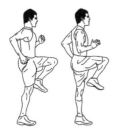

10 march steps

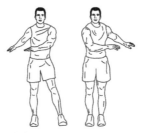

20 side-to-side steps

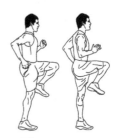

10 march steps

17   Cardio Rock Workout

Raising your game in the cardio stakes is easy. All you need to do is to load large muscle groups quickly, ask them to perform under pressure and give them just enough time to recover before you ask them to do it all again. The Cardio Rock workout utilizes relatively few exercises in quick succession to achieve just that. Get into the sweat zone and feel your muscles heating up and your body burning at a high level as you go through one exercise after another in quick succession with the Cardio Rock workout.

Cardio Rock

DAREBEE WORKOUT © darebee.com

LEVEL I 3 sets **LEVEL II** 5 sets **LEVEL III** 7 sets **REST** up to 2 minutes

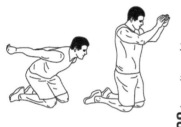

20 kneeling skiers

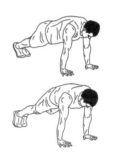

10 plank with lateral thrusts

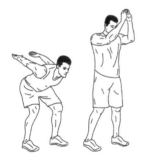

20 half squat skiers

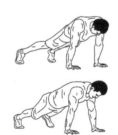

10 wide leg plank with lateral thrusts

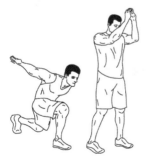

20 reverse lunge skiers

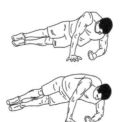

10 side plank thrusts

18 Chase Workout

When you're being chased you need to run. Your body requires strong muscles, powerful tendons, a cardiovascular system that will really get your heart pumping and your blood flowing to all the right muscle groups, plus you need your aerobic performance, your VO2 Max volume to be as near as optimal as possible. Chase does all of that, plus, since the difference between chasing and being chased is separated by a hair's breadth, it really prepares you for the times when you will need to be the one doing the chasing.

Make it harder. When doing flutter kicks keep your chin on your chest and make it a little harder on your abs.

CHASE

DAREBEE WORKOUT © darebee.com

LEVEL I 3 sets **LEVEL II** 5 sets **LEVEL III** 7 sets **REST** up to 2 minutes

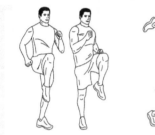
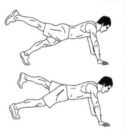
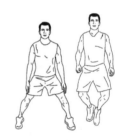

3combos: 10 high knees + 4 plank leg raises   **10** hop heel clicks

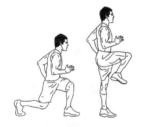
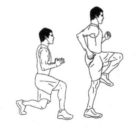
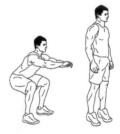

10combos successive lunge step-ups   **10** squat calf raises

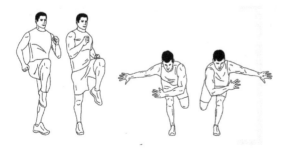
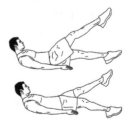

3combos: 10 high knees + 4 side-to-side hops   **40** flutter kicks

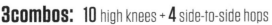

19   Chisel Workout

Getting that chiseled physique requires patience, perseverance and the ability to put in the time one day after another. Chisel, of course, is the workout that'll help you do all this. A combination of aerobic and strength exercises it works all the major muscle groups so that your body keeps on changing the way you want it to.

Make it harder: Two minutes rest time is way too much. Make it half that and feel your aerobic.

CHISEL

DAREBEE WORKOUT © darebee.com

LEVEL I 3 sets **LEVEL II** 5 sets **LEVEL III** 7 sets **REST** up to 2 minutes

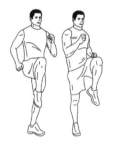

20 high knees

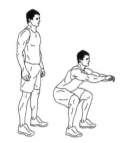

10 squats

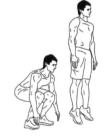

10 jump squats

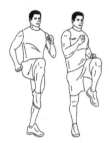

20 high knees

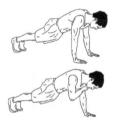

10 shoulder taps

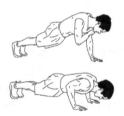

10 shoulder tap push-ups

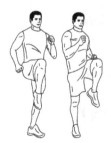

20 high knees

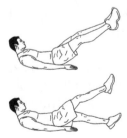

10 flutter kicks

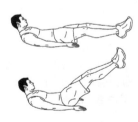

10 leg raises

20 Contender Workout

One of the hardest things you can do is get into a ring and go a few rounds. Beyond the fact that there is the inevitable exchange of blows you are pushing your entire body to the limit with no room to ease off, no matter how much your muscles ache or your lungs burn. As a physical test the Contender takes you through one exercise after another, slowly loading each muscle group and then asking you to exercise even as fatigue tags at you. Well, there is no exchange of blows taking place, so dig deep and feel the burn.

Make it harder: Work to complete each exercise as fast as possible without compromising the quality of the technique. This will help load your aerobic performance helping you feel the aerobic load boxers feel in the ring.

CONTENDER

DAREBEE WORKOUT © darebee.com
LEVEL I 3 sets **LEVEL II** 5 sets **LEVEL III** 7 sets **REST** up to 2 minutes

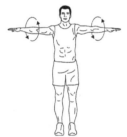

30 bounces

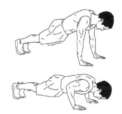

5 push-ups

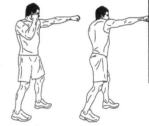

30 punches

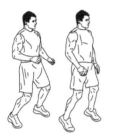

30 arm rotations

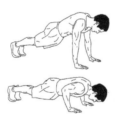

5 push-ups

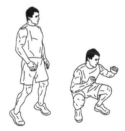

30 squats

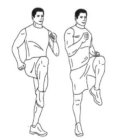

30 high knees

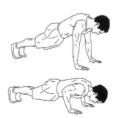

5 push-ups

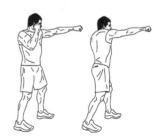

30 punches

21   Dash Workout

Building up speed relies on forcing muscles to undergo a few adaptive changes. There are two parts to becoming lightning-fast, the first part requires developing the muscle structure itself, increasing the number of neurons and developing fast-twitch action fiber. The second part requires strengthening of all the supporting muscle groups and tendons that help major muscle groups perform. The DASH workout is designed to help you develop both. Each exercise is performed at full speed.

Make it harder. Reduce rest time to one minute for a full challenge to your aerobic performance.

Dash

DAREBEE WORKOUT © darebee.com

LEVEL I 3 sets **LEVEL II** 5 sets **LEVEL III** 7 sets **REST** up to 2 minutes

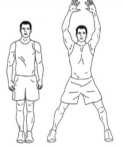

20 jumping jacks

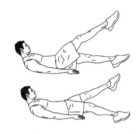

10 flutter kicks

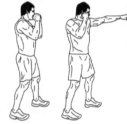

40 punches

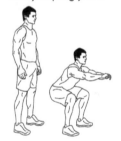

20 squats

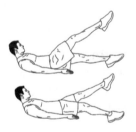

10 flutter kicks

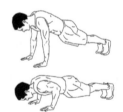

10 push-ups

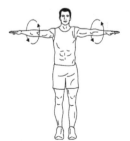

40 raised arm circles

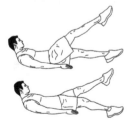

10 flutter kicks

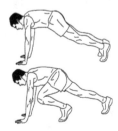

10 climbers

22 DNA:Rewrite Workout

What if you could transform yourself into the kind of physically capable person you want to be? How would you rewrite your DNA? This is a workout that helps you explore the possibilities lying at the boundaries of your capabilities.

Make it better. When you're doing lunge step-ups lean your upper body back so your abs come into play, balance your center of gravity over your hips and that creates a dynamic stress position that also works your hamstrings, lower back and glutes with each knee raise.

DNA:rewrite

DAREBEE WORKOUT © darebee.com

LEVEL I 3 sets **LEVEL II** 5 sets **LEVEL III** 7 sets **REST** up to 2 minutes

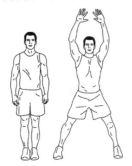

20 jumping jacks

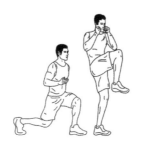

20 lunge step-ups

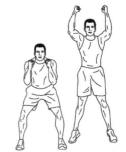

20 jumps

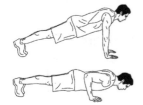

10 push-ups

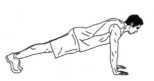

10-count plank

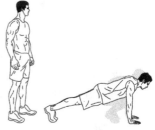

10 basic burpees

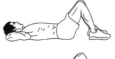

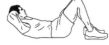

10 crunches

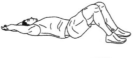

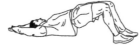

10 bridges

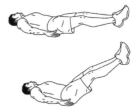

10 leg raises

23   Extractor Workout

There are some days when all you want to do is go through a workout where you do not have to think much, or concentrate hard. You take yourself out of the picture and let your body do its thing. The Extractor workout is just the thing that will do that for you.

Make it better: When performing jumping lunges clear the floor by at least a foot each time, upping the pressure on your quads.

EXTRACTOR

DAREBEE WORKOUT © darebee.com

LEVEL I 3 sets **LEVEL II** 5 sets **LEVEL III** 7 sets **REST** up to 2 minutes

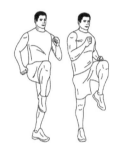

20 high knees

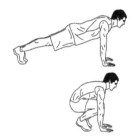

5 plank jump-ins

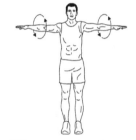

20 raised arm circles

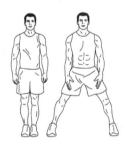

20 half jacks

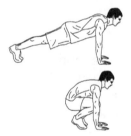

5 plank jump-ins

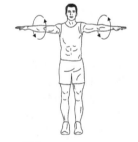

20 raised arm circles

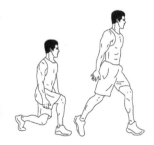

20 jumping lunges

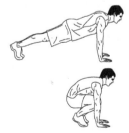

5 plank jump-ins

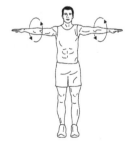

20 raised arm circles

24 Forge Workout

Some workouts make you sweat and some others get you started on the journey to forge yourself into the best version of you, you can be. The Forge workout is definitely one of the latter. Combining fast moving cardio exercises with body combat moves it tasks major muscle groups to move gracefully, under pressure. Add some solid core work and an eccentric/isometric challenge at the end and you end up with a great way to shape your body in the way you want it to.

Make it better: Perform all standing moves on the balls of your feet.

THE FORGE

DAREBEE WORKOUT © darebee.com

LEVEL I 3 sets **LEVEL II** 5 sets **LEVEL III** 7 sets **REST** up to 2 minutes

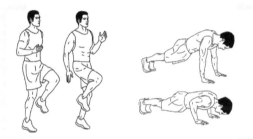

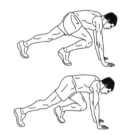

3combos: **10** high knees + **2** push-ups

10 climbers

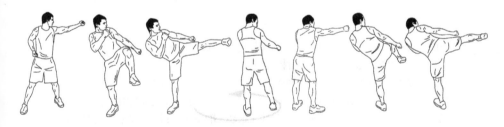

10 combos backfist + side kick + hop & rotate + backfist + side kick

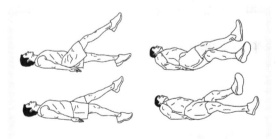

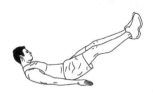

3combos: **10** flutter kicks + **2** scissors

10-count raised leg hold

25 Heist Workout

Some workouts are chosen and some workouts choose you. If you're doing The Heist workout you will see what that means. There is an overlap between anaerobic and aerobic work, concentric and eccentric muscle movement and isometric core work when you're already tired. Of course you know what you need for Heist, right? Great speed, splendid reactions, stamina, strength, focus, a little aerobic capacity and excellent recovery time. Get in. Get Out. What can possibly go wrong?

Make it harder: You can't. Yep, you heard right.

THE HEIST

Get in. Get out. What can go wrong?

DAREBEE WORKOUT
© darebee.com
LEVEL I 3 sets
LEVEL II 5 sets
LEVEL III 7 sets
REST up to 2 minutes

HIGH BURN

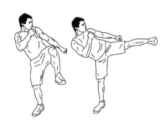

10combos: **1** squat + **2** double side kicks

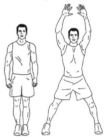

10 jumping jacks

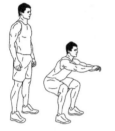

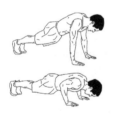

10combos: **1** push-ups + **4** punches

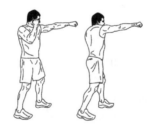

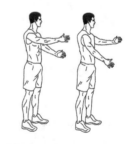

10 scissor chops

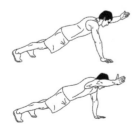

10 plank arm raises

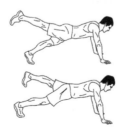

10 plank leg raises

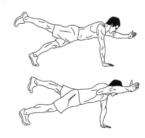

10 plank alt arm/ leg raises

26   Hell Raider Workout

For days when you need a light, fast, energizing workout, Hell Raider delivers the goods. It won't burn your lungs, desiccate your body or make your muscles scream but it will get your body moving, your heart pumping and your lungs working which is always a win.

Extra Credit: Add some extra weight. Try a weighted vest (if you want to go hardcore on this) or light ankle weights.

Hell Raider

DAREBEE WORKOUT © darebee.com

LEVEL I 3 sets **LEVEL II** 5 sets **LEVEL III** 7 sets **REST** up to 2 minutes

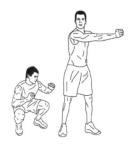

20 squat + side chop

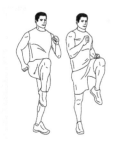

4combos: **10** high knees + **2** jump knee tucks

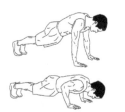

10 push-ups

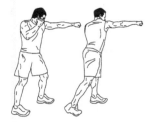 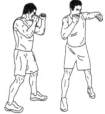

4combos: **10** punches + **2** hooks

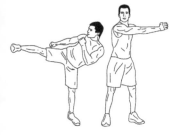

20 side kick + side chop

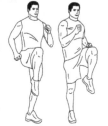

4combos: **10** high knees + **2** side-to-side jumps

27   Jacks Workout

Some workouts are just designed to put emphasis on "work". Without work there can be no change. Without change there can be no improvement. And improvement there shall be with the Jacks Pyramid workout. 'Nuff said.

Make it better: Never let your heels touch the ground. Perform the entire workout on the balls of your feet.

JACKS PYRAMID

DAREBEE WORKOUT © darebee.com

LEVEL I 3 sets **LEVEL II** 5 sets **LEVEL III** 7 sets **REST** up to 2 minutes

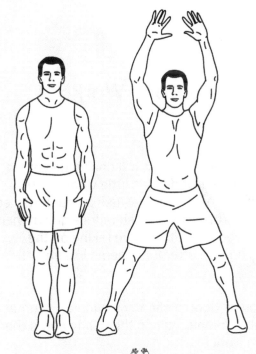

10 jumping jacks

10-count rest

15 jumping jacks

10-count rest

20 jumping jacks

10-count rest

25 jumping jacks

10-count rest

20 jumping jacks

10-count rest

15 jumping jacks

10-count rest

10 jumping jacks

**LOW IMPACT
ALTERNATIVE
STEP JACKS**

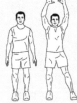

28 Power Burpee Workout

Burpees are one of those exercises that will challenge you no matter how fit you are. To break it down a little what you're doing is pitting yourself against the planet, using your muscles to fight the pull of gravity. This is why it can reduce grown men to tears. It does also give you results. You're taking on the planet. All of it! Everything else after that seems like an anti-climax.

Make it better. Consciously tighten slightly your lower stomach, flattening your lower abdominals, pulling them in towards the spine and making them work harder.

POWER BURPEE

start   finish

DAREBEE WORKOUT
© darebee.com
6 reps each | 3 sets
up to 2 minutes
rest between sets

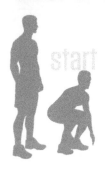

1
raised leg
push-up

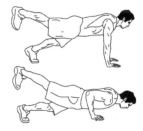

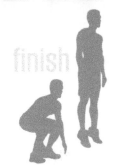

2
shoulder taps
each side

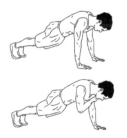

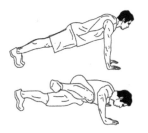

3
push-up
side crunch
each side

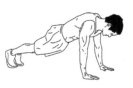

4
10-count
plank hold

29   Quick Silver Workout

Move faster without stressing your joints with the Quicksilver workout. It helps you develop muscle stability and mobility almost by stealth, its exercises are perfect for that indoor workout on days when you have a sofa handy.

Make it better: When marching raise your knees to waist height.

QUICK
SiLVER

DAREBEE WORKOUT
© darebee.com
LEVEL I 3 sets
LEVEL II 5 sets
LEVEL III 7 sets
REST up to 2 minutes

HIGH BURN

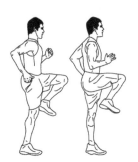
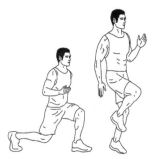
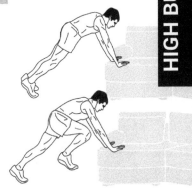
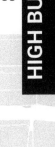

20 march steps

20 lunge step-ups

20 incline slow climbers

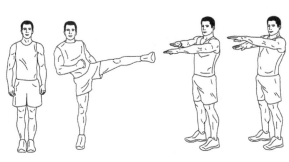
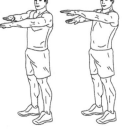
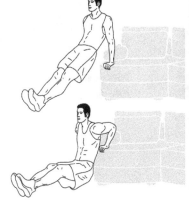

10 side leg raises

10 arm scissors

10 tricep dips

30 Rebel Workout

Rebels acknowledge no rules which means they have to be ready for anything. Our Rebel workout prepares you for almost anything. Its combination of static and ballistic exercises puts your body through its paces in a way that says "I am really preparing to break the rules".

Make it harder: Cut down rest time between sets to just 60 seconds and push your aerobic performance.

REBEL

DAREBEE WORKOUT
ⓒ darebee.com
LEVEL I 3 sets
LEVEL II 5 sets
LEVEL III 7 sets
REST up to 2 minutes

HIGH BURN

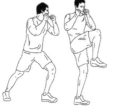
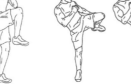
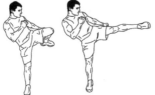
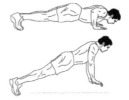

40 knee strikes   **40** turning kicks   **10** power push-ups

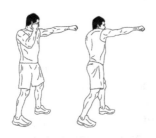
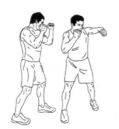
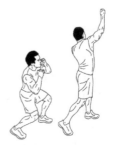

20combos jab + jab + cross + hook + upper cut

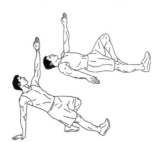
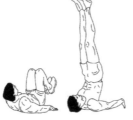
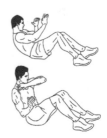

10 get-ups   **10** butt-ups   **10** elbow strike sit-ups

31 Reboot Workout

Reboot your body, mind and spirit with the Reboot workout designed to get you moving, your arms and legs pumping and your heart thumping. If that sounds like a lot of hard work it is because it is exactly that. The alternating fast/slow tempo segments work the muscles both ballistically and isometrically, forcing your body to work even when it should be resting which means the muscles are truly tested. Dive in and feel the benefits.

Make it harder: Clear the floor by at least a foot every time you jump during Burpees.

R=BOOT

DAREBEE WORKOUT © darebee.com

LEVEL I 3 sets **LEVEL II** 5 sets **LEVEL III** 7 sets **REST** up to 2 minutes

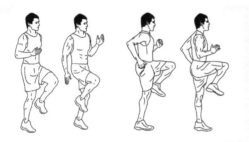

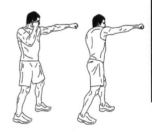

3combos: **20** high knees + **10** march   **40** punches

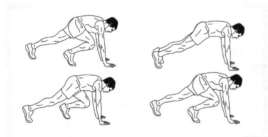

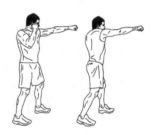

3combos: **20** climbers + **10** slow climbers   **40** punches

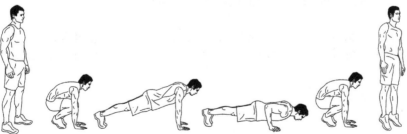

10 burpees (squat + plank + push-up + jump-in + jump up)

32   Roaster Workout

Getting your muscles to the point where you can practically feel the heat coming off them gives the sentence "going for the burn" an entirely new meaning altogether. The Roaster workout helps you attack some major muscle groups again and again from one exercise to another, varying the load, movement and intensity while still engaging the muscles. You will feel your body's temperature rise and you will feel the burn and after it's all over you should feel positively roasted.

Make it harder: Reduce rest time between sets to just 60 seconds and feel the burn in your lings as well as your muscles.

THE ROASTER

DAREBEE WORKOUT © darebee.com

LEVEL I 3 sets **LEVEL II** 5 sets **LEVEL III** 7 sets **REST** up to 2 minutes

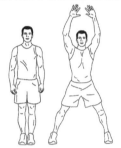

20 jumping jacks

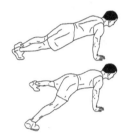

2 plank jacks

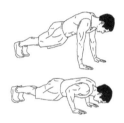

2 push-ups (fast!)

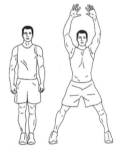

20 jumping jacks

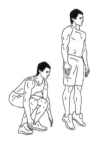

2 jump squats

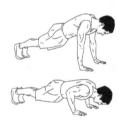

2 push-ups (fast!)

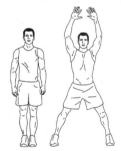

20 jumping jacks

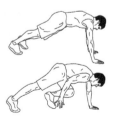

2 climber taps

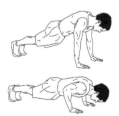

2 push-ups (fast!)

33 Scout Workout

Scouts are fast on their feet and strong enough to take on anything. The Scout workout works on speed, strength and power to deliver an all-round body experience. The change between normal sets and fast sets pushes muscles to work harder and faster helping you make gains in a very short time.

Make it better. Go really fast on fast high knees helping your aerobic system feel the load.

Scout

DAREBEE WORKOUT
© darebee.com
LEVEL I 3 sets
LEVEL II 5 sets
LEVEL III 7 sets
REST up to 2 minutes

HIGH BURN

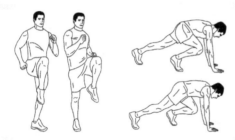

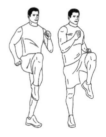

4combos: **10** high knees + **4** climbers

40 fast high knees

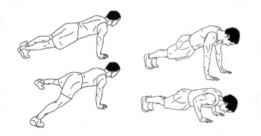

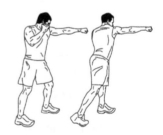

4combos: **10** plank jacks + **4** push-ups

40 fast punches

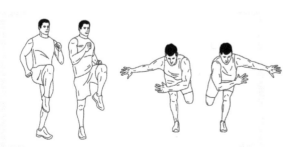

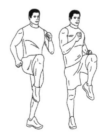

4combos: **10** high knees + **4** side-to-side jumps

40 fast high knees

34   Skier Workout

There is more than one way to train skier muscles. Balance, control, coordination, these are all skills that can be developed using specific exercises and the Skier workout allows you to do just that even if you happen to be living in the tropics. All you need to do then is find a quiet place, give yourself just a little room and some time and let the Skier workout begin to transform your body.

skier

DAREBEE WORKOUT © darebee.com

5 sets | up to 2 minute rest between sets

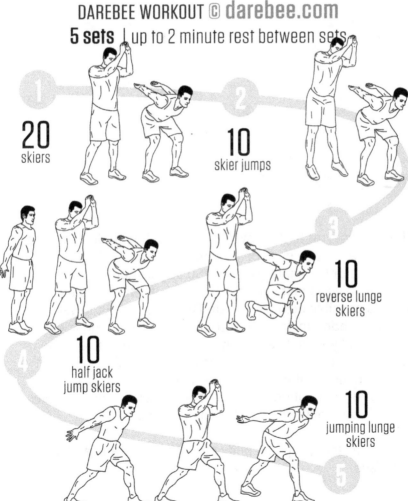

20 skiers

10 skier jumps

10 reverse lunge skiers

10 half jack jump skiers

10 jumping lunge skiers

35   Spy Workout

There is a secret to the Spy Workout that has to do with core muscles and body control. Whether you're doing half jacks or plan jacks or backfists (with an 180 degree hop) or sideckicks, your feet always just skim the floor. You try to spend as little time as possible being in the air. That means your lower abs and core abdominals come into play, your pelvic muscles are key and your side and front hip flexors are crucial. You learn to exercise total body control in a dynamic movement environment. Ok, it may not quite make you a spy, but it will make you aware of how you move and the way your muscles control your body, which is a pretty cool thing.

Make it better: Keep you body straight in all plank and bodysaw exercises.

Spy

DAREBEE WORKOUT © darebee.com

LEVEL I 3 sets **LEVEL II** 5 sets **LEVEL III** 7 sets **REST** up to 2 minutes

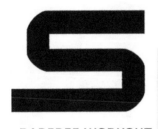

20 half jacks

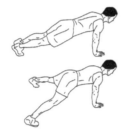

10 plank jacks

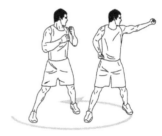

20 bounce + backfist

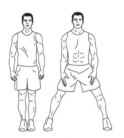

20 high knees

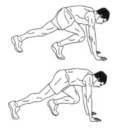

10 climbers

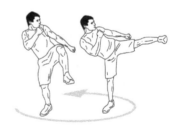

20 bounce + side kick

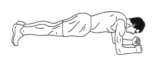

10-count plank

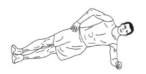

10-count side plank

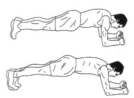

10 bodysaw

36 Torch Workout

Torch your day and your stamina with a fast-paced, jaunty workout that will light up your day and make your body feel more alive than it has any right to be. The Torch workout is the kind of thing you want your day to end on or your week to begin with but it's perfect as a workout any time you want to simply feel your body moving and your blood pumping.

Make it better: During side leg raises bring your leg to waist height, knees straight.

TORCH

DAREBEE WORKOUT © darebee.com

LEVEL I 3 sets **LEVEL II** 5 sets **LEVEL III** 7 sets **REST** up to 2 minutes

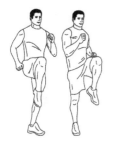

20 high knees

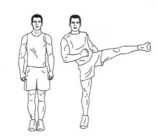

20 side leg raises

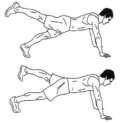

10 plank leg raises

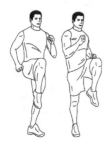

20 high knees

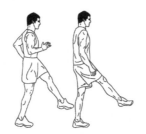

20 straight leg bounds

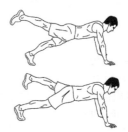

10 plank leg raises

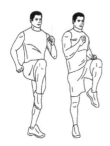

20 high knees

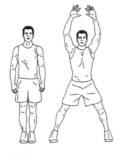

20 jumping jacks

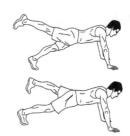

10 plank leg raises

37   Ultimate Burn Workout

A little burn goes a long way. And some movement can produce a whole lot of burn if it's constant and does not let up. The Ultimate Burn workout requires non-stop movement, you're on the balls of your feet, all the time jumping, bouncing, twisting, hoping. As your calves begin to feel the strain your lungs will also begin to feel the load which means you're doing everything just the way it should be done.

Make it harder. Reduce rest time to just 90 seconds to really put the strain on your system to recover fast.

Ultimate Burn

DAREBEE WORKOUT © darebee.com

LEVEL I 3 sets **LEVEL II** 5 sets **LEVEL III** 7 sets **REST** up to 2 minutes

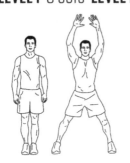

20 jumping jacks

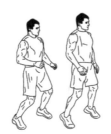

20 bounces

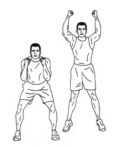

10 jumps

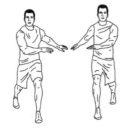

20 twist jacks

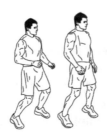

20 bounces

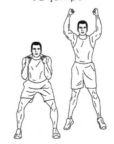

10 jumps

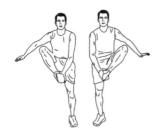

20 toe tap hops

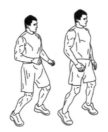

20 bounces

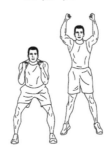

10 jumps

38   Aim to Misbehave Workout

Making mischief requires stamina and stamina needs strength and strength needs muscles to work after they are loaded to the point of being fatigued, all of which brings us to the I Aim To Misbehave workout that takes your upper body strength and transforms it into a mischief-making engine. You just need to go deep and keep your body straight in the push ups and really throw those punches out to see exactly what all this means.

I aim to misbehave

DAREBEE WORKOUT © darebee.com

LEVEL I 3 sets **LEVEL II** 4 sets **LEVEL III** 5 sets **REST** up to 2 minutes

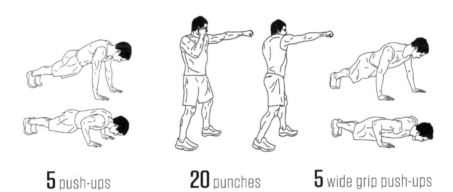

5 push-ups   **20** punches   **5** wide grip push-ups

STRENGTH

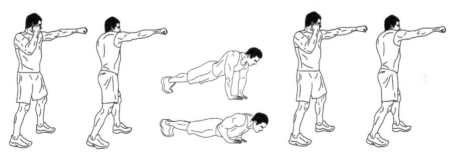

20 punches   **5** close grip push-ups   **20** punches

39   Armageddon Workout

You have two arms which means you will be experiencing twice the joy as this workout uses the rapid motion of the arms to also challenge the core and abs and even your glutes and quads and hamstrings. The amazing thing about the connected body is that the upper body powers the lower body so strong arms help you run faster, longer and the lower body powers the upper one so that strong legs help you punch harder.

Make it harder: Make the scissors blindingly fast, blurring the motion of your arms. Not only does it activate your abs but it also challenges your hand-eye coordination.

ARMAGEDDON

DAREBEE WORKOUT © darebee.com

LEVEL I 3 sets **LEVEL II** 5 sets **LEVEL III** 7 sets **REST** up to 2 minutes

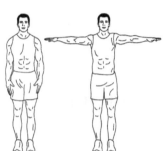

20 side arm raises

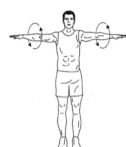

20 raised arm circles

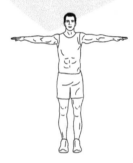

20-count arm hold

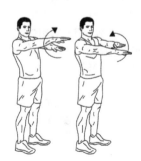

20 fast scissors

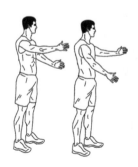

20 scissor chops

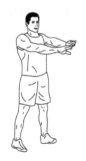

20-count arm hold

40   Arms of Steel Workout

Whatever sport you may be doing, your arms are a critical component of it and the stronger they are, the better you get. Getting them strong however is not an easy job. This is where the Arms of Steel workout comes in. Not only does it tackle your arms from practically every angle but it also gives you no rest time, forcing your muscles to recover on the fly. Afterwards not only will you have arms of steel, you will also have the kind of arms that can power, manned, winged flight, almost.

Make it harder: Work fast but hard, pulling your punches back as fast as you send them out, working both the agonist and antagonist muscles.

Arms of Steel

DAREBEE WORKOUT © darebee.com

LEVEL I 3 sets **LEVEL II** 4 sets **LEVEL III** 5 sets **REST** up to 2 minutes

STRENGTH

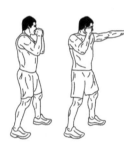

10 push-ups

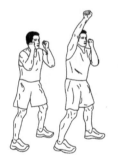

20 punches

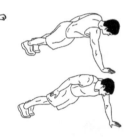

10 thigh taps

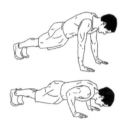

10 shoulder taps

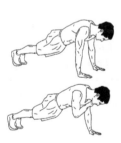

20 overhead punches

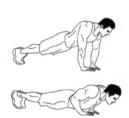

10 tricep push-ups

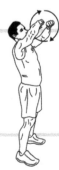

2 minutes rotating punches
aka speed bag punches
instead of complete rest after every set,
at any speed

41 Bodyguard Workout

Endurance is the capability of muscles to work long as well as hard. Like any athletic skill it can be developed. The Bodyguard workout helps you develop the ability to do sustained, high-energy work, long after everyone else around you has dropped to the ground with exhaustion.

Make it better: When performing high knees bring your knees to waist height.

BODYGUARD

DAREBEE WORKOUT © darebee.com

LEVEL I 3 sets **LEVEL II** 5 sets **LEVEL III** 7 sets **REST** up to 2 minutes

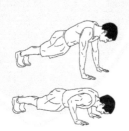

20 push-ups

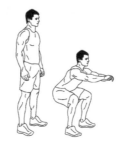

40 squats

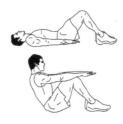

40 sit-ups

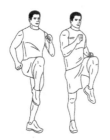

40 high knees

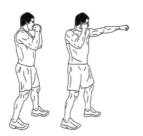

40 punches

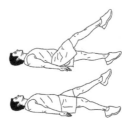

40 flutter kicks

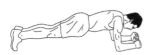

20sec plank

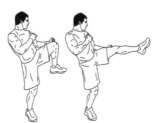

40 front kicks

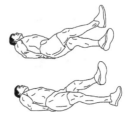

40 scissors

42   Body Hack Workout

We train because what we really want to do is hack our bodies. Control them. make them vehicles that do our bidding. That's never easy. It takes time, effort, hard work. The Body Hack workout is a step towards that direction: controlling the body you live in. If there ever was a rinse, apply, repeat formula that produced the desirable outcome, this would come pretty close to being it.

Make it harder: When doing fast push ups inhale on the way down and exhale on the way up, using your abs to add to your going up speed for a harder workout.

BODY HACK

DAREBEE WORKOUT © darebee.com

LEVEL I 3 sets **LEVEL II** 5 sets **LEVEL III** 7 sets **REST** up to 2 minutes

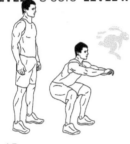

10 fast squats

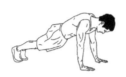

10-count plank

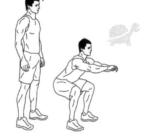

10 slow squats

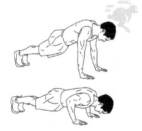

5 fast push-ups

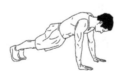

10-count plank

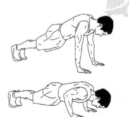

5 slow push-ups

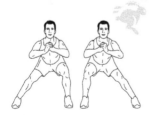

10 fast side-to-side lunges

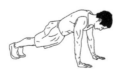

10-count plank

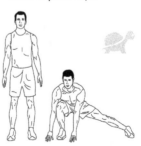

10 slow side lunges

43 Bootcamp Workout

When you start the Bootcamp workout you realize just why it's called Bootcamp. Each exercise is designed to build on the previous one, testing strength and endurance, balance and stability, coordination and technique. With overlapping muscles working, this becomes the kind of workout you know your body will know it did the day after.

Make it harder: Slow the push ups down engaging more of your muscle fibers as you go up and down.

BOOTCAMP

DAREBEE WORKOUT © darebee.com

LEVEL I 3 sets **LEVEL II** 5 sets **LEVEL III** 7 sets **REST** up to 2 minutes

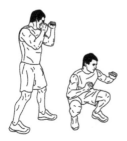

20 squats

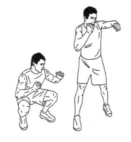

20 squat + hook

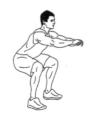

20-count squat hold

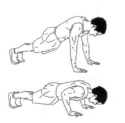

10 push-ups

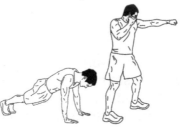

10 plank step-out + punches

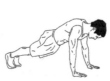

10-count plank

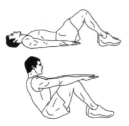

10 sit-ups

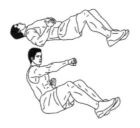

10 sit-up + punches

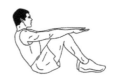

10-count sit-up hold

44 Boss Fight Workout

A Boss Fight needs to be savored (which is why there are ten sets). It needs strength, stamina, grit. The kind of spirit that does not back down. In return it trains almost every muscle group in the body using concentric and dynamic movements. It helps build up endurance but it's the strength component that should get you excited, plus it is a Boss Fight. No backing down, now.

Make it better: When performing Squat Hold Punches make sure your legs are at a 90 degree angle.

BOSS FIGHT

DAREBEE WORKOUT © darebee.com

1 bar = 1 set **rest between sets** up to 2 minutes

STRENGTH

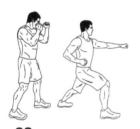

20 lunge punches

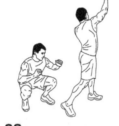

20 squat + uppercut

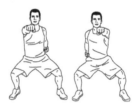

20 squat hold punches

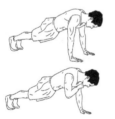

10 shoulder taps

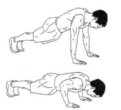

10 push-ups

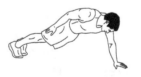

10-count one-arm plank

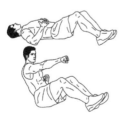

10 sit-up punches

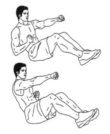

10 sitting punches

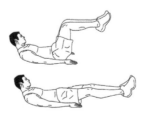

10 crunch kicks

45   Boulder Workout

Strength is not just about muscle size. It depends on muscle density, the type of muscle fiber you have. The composition of each bundle of muscle and its ability to perform under physical stress. The Boulder workout definitely creates some physical stress to challenge the muscles so you get to feel like a rock.

Make it better: When performing raised-leg push ups keep your raised leg completely straight at the knee.

THE BOULDER

DAREBEE WORKOUT © darebee.com

LEVEL I 3 sets **LEVEL II** 5 sets **LEVEL III** 7 sets **REST** up to 2 minutes

STRENGTH

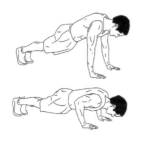

10 push-ups

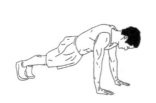

10-count plank

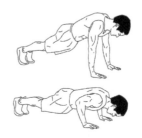

10 push-ups

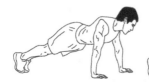

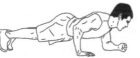

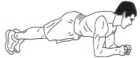

10 up and down planks

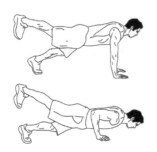

10 raised leg push-ups

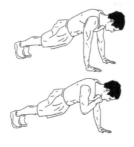

10 shoulder taps

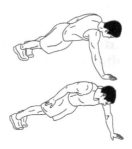

10 thigh taps

46   Bounty Hunter Workout

There is an easy way to make a workout hard: alternate between static and ballistic movements, loading the muscles with bodyweight and then asking them to explode and move through their full range of motion when they are already tired. If that sounds a tad hard it is because, it is. It is also highly effective delivering a high-burn body-shaping workout you really feel working five minutes in.

Extra Credit: Pick up the speed of your punches immediately after push ups.

BOUNTY HUNTER

DAREBEE WORKOUT
© darebee.com
LEVEL I 3 sets
LEVEL II 5 sets
LEVEL III 7 sets
REST up to 2 minutes

STRENGTH

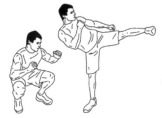

20 squat + side kick

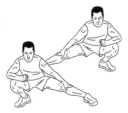

4 side-to-side lunges

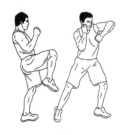

20 knee strike + elbow strike

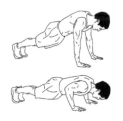
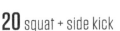

20 push-ups

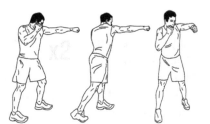

20 jab + jab + cross + hook

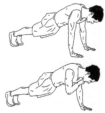

20 shoulder taps

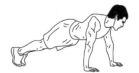

10 up and down planks   +

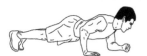
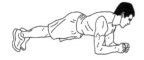

10-count elbow plank hold finish

47 Boxer Workout

Boxers have blazingly-fast hands, incredible stamina, focus, strength, perseverance, the ability to compartmentalize pain and great spatial awareness. All of which can now be yours provided you use this workout to remake your body and transform your spirit. Plus, when you next hear the Rocky soundtrack you'll be able to deservedly throw your arms up towards the sky and jog on the spot (com'on, you know you want to).

Tip: When performing push-ups keep your body perfectly straight and your abs tight so you also work the abdominal wall.

BOXER

5 SETS DAREBEE WORKOUT © darebee.com
up to 2 minutes rest between rounds

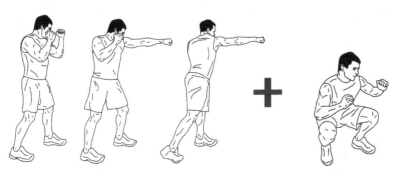

5 minute shadow boxing   **every 30 seconds** double squat

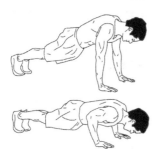
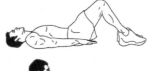
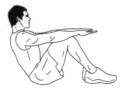

push-ups
level I 5 reps
level II 10 reps
level III 15 reps

sit-ups
level I 10 reps
level II 20 reps
level III 30 reps

48   Centurion Workout

In the ancient world fitness was a necessity rather than a pastime. The Centurion workout aims at functional fitness targeting the muscles used by the body when it needs to move fast, jump far and fight.

Make it better. When performing the Jab + Cross combination twist on the balls of your feet and throw your body weight behind the punch.

CENTURION

DAREBEE WORKOUT © darebee.com

LEVEL I 3 sets **LEVEL II** 5 sets **LEVEL III** 7 sets **REST** up to 2 minutes

STRENGTH

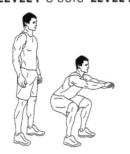

10combo squat + calf raise

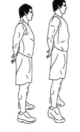

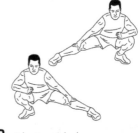

10 side-to-side lunges

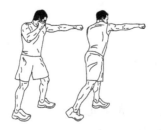

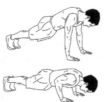

10combo jab + cross + push-up

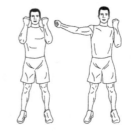

10 side-to-side backfists

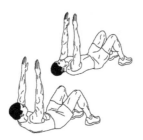

10 high crunches

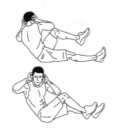

10 knee-to-elbow crunches

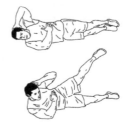

10 side jackknives

49 Combat Strength Workout

Turn your body into a pillar of strength, capable of almost anything with the Combat Strength workout. As the name suggests the aim is to challenge major muscle groups building up the strength and speed you'd need in a hypothetical combat scenario where all you have is your body and the razor-sharp mind that guides it.

Make it better: Speed up everything raising the body's thermic response and getting to the aerobic part of the workout faster.

Combat Strength

DAREBEE WORKOUT © darebee.com

LEVEL I 3 sets **LEVEL II** 5 sets **LEVEL III** 7 sets **REST** up to 2 minutes

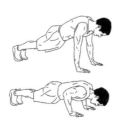

10 push-ups

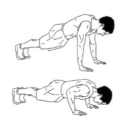

10combos push-up + jab + cross

STRENGTH

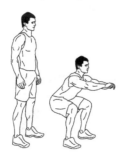

10 squats

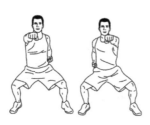

40 squat hold punches

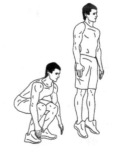

10 jump squats

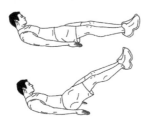

20 leg raises

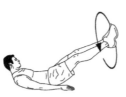

20 raised leg circles

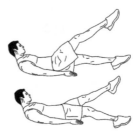

20 flutter kicks

50 Commando Workout

There are times when what you want is your body to obey you, explicitly. You want your muscles to respond quickly and with precision. The Commando workout pushes all the right buttons, helping your body develop the kind of precision control you've been looking for.

Make it better: Work your speed bag punches at above eye level and reverse the direction every few punches so that you go both clockwise in your rotations and anti-clockwise.

COMMANDO

DAREBEE WORKOUT © darebee.com

LEVEL I 3 sets **LEVEL II** 4 sets **LEVEL III** 5 sets **REST** up to 2 minutes

STRENGTH

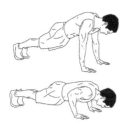

to failure push-ups

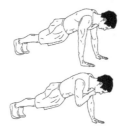

10 shoulder taps

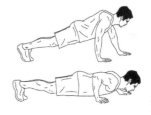

4 staggered push-ups

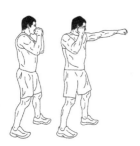

40 punches

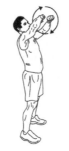

40 speed bag punches

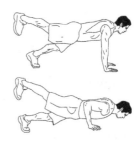

4 raised leg push-ups

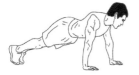

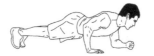

10 up and down planks

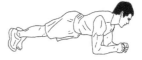

51   Crucible Workout

For those who have played Destiny once or twice, the Crucible is a place where Guardians go to test their skills and cement their reputations. This Crucible is a little different, no skills or armor will be gained by doing the workout but your reputation might well be cemented.

Make it better: With each lunge make sure the knee of your back leg touches the floor, for a really deep execution of the technique.

CRUCIBLE

DAREBEE WORKOUT © darebee.com

LEVEL I 4 push-ups **LEVEL II** 8 push-ups **LEVEL III** 10 push-ups
LEVEL I 3 sets **LEVEL II** 5 sets **LEVEL III** 7 sets **REST** up to 2 minutes

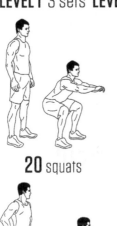

20 squats

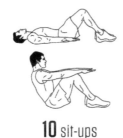

10 sit-ups

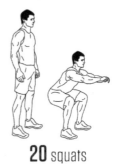

20 squats

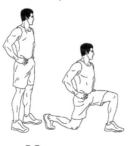

20 lunges

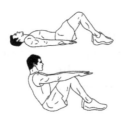

10 sit-ups

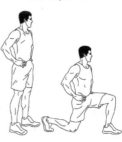

20 lunges

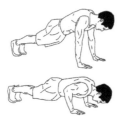

X push-ups

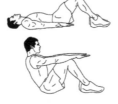

10 sit-ups

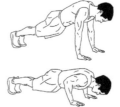

X push-ups

52 Dragon Slayer Workout

If you're really intent on taking on dragons you'd better focus on your physical fitness and make sure it's up to scratch otherwise your dragon-slaying career will be kinda shortlived. The Dragon Slayer workout makes sure you don't fail just coz you weren't strong enough.

Make it better. Add some wrist and ankle weights for that extra special burn.

DRAGON SLAYER

DAREBEE WORKOUT © darebee.com

LEVEL I 3 sets **LEVEL II** 5 sets **LEVEL III** 7 sets **REST** up to 2 minutes

STRENGTH

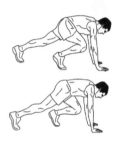

20 climbers

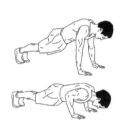

6 push-ups

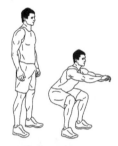

6 squats

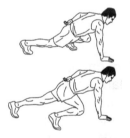

20 one arm climbers

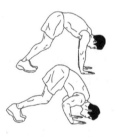

6 pike push-ups

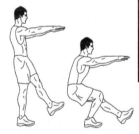

6 pistol squats

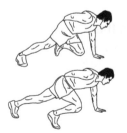

20 one arm climbers

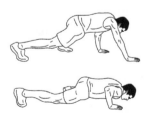

6 dragon push-ups

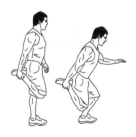

6 shrimp squats

53 Equalizer Workout

When you are a one-man army, with a penchant for optimizing your every move to achieve that perfection of balance and power you know that the exercises that will take you there have to do with muscle control. The Equalizer workout may not quite turn you into a deadly weapon but it will give you the control you crave to have over your body, provided you do the sets enough times.

Make it better: Slow down your push-ups forcing the muscles to fire longer, under heavier load, providing better results.

EQUALIZER

DAREBEE WORKOUT © darebee.com

LEVEL I 3 sets **LEVEL II** 5 sets **LEVEL III** 7 sets **REST** up to 2 minutes

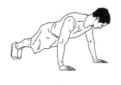

10 push-ups

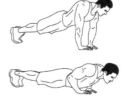

4 wide grip push-ups

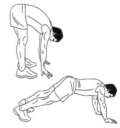

4 close grip push-ups

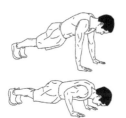

10 reverse flutter kicks

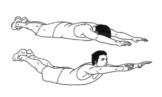

10 superman stretches

4 plank walk-outs

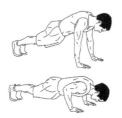

10 push-ups

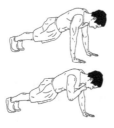

4 shoulder taps

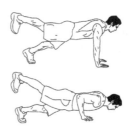

4 raised leg push-ups

54 Fremen Workout

When you're destined to be amongst the best fighters in the Universe from birth, physical fitness is a way of life. The Spice will make that life long but just how awesome it will be is entirely down to you. Life on the desert planet is naturally harsh. The environment demands strength, endurance and the ability to survive and succeed on relatively few resources. Muscles have to justify every gram of their existence so there is no point having bulk when what you really need is strength. This is a workout worthy of a Sandworm Rider. Designed to build up core strength and dense muscle it's just the ticket for those whom Shai Hulud favors.

Tip: To increase muscle density and promote greater strength with less bulk perform the wide grip push-ups to a slow count of ten on the way down and a slow count of ten on the way up.

FREMEN

DAREBEE WORKOUT © darebee.com

LEVEL I 3 sets **LEVEL II** 5 sets **LEVEL III** 7 sets **REST** up to 2 minutes

STRENGTH

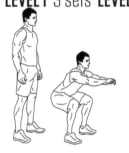

10 squats

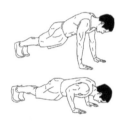

5 push-ups

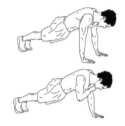

10 shoulder taps

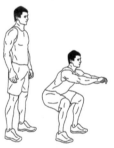

10 squats

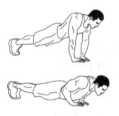

5 close grip push-ups

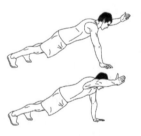

10 plank arm raises

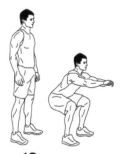

10 squats

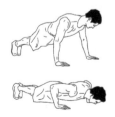

5 wide grip push-ups

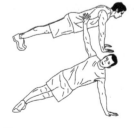

10 planks with rotations

55 Gambit Workout

If you had really strong legs and a powerful core you would be able to synchronize your upper and lower body muscles in a way that would totally transform the way you move. The Gambit is there to make sure that your lower body and core are worked in a fashion that provides the foundation for just this kind of synchronization.

Make it better: Go deep in your squats and hold your body absolutely straight when holding the plank.

GAMBIT

DAREBEE WORKOUT © darebee.com

LEVEL I 3 sets **LEVEL II** 5 sets **LEVEL III** 7 sets **REST** up to 2 minutes

STRENGTH

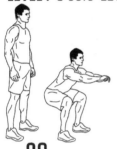

20 squats

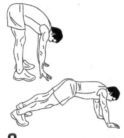

6 plank walk-outs

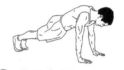

10-count plank hold

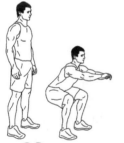

20 squats

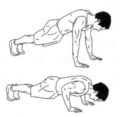

6 slow push-ups

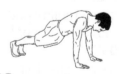

10-count plank hold

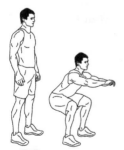

20 squats

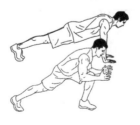

6 plank-into-lunges

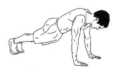

10-count plank hold

56   Gladiator Workout

Gladiators were fierce people. To survive they required good core stability and strength followed by excellent ballistic movement capability. If you're ready to leap into the arena and battle to the death, for the glory of combat, then this workout is a good way to prepare.

Tip: This is a workout for strength and endurance. There is no rest between the exercises so make sure you maintain the intensity of your performance.

GLADIATOR

DAREBEE WORKOUT © darebee.com

LEVEL I 3 sets **LEVEL II** 5 sets **LEVEL III** 7 sets **REST** up to 2 minutes

STRENGTH

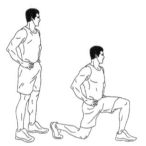

40 lunges

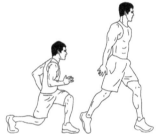

20 jumping lunges

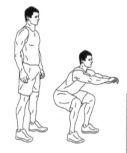

20 squats

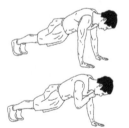

20 shoulder taps

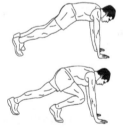

40 slow climbers

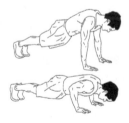

10 push-ups

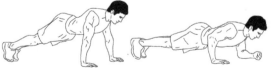
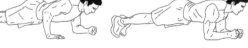

10 up & down planks

57   Golem Workout

If you're a mythical creature that's unstoppable you need the kind of basic strength and core power that renders you a force of nature. The Golem workout takes you back to basics for a reason. It really helps you take your core fitness to the level you need.

Make it better: When performing jump squats and jumping lunges try to clear the floor, each time, by at least 1ft.

GOLEM

DAREBEE WORKOUT © **darebee.com**

LEVEL I 3 sets **LEVEL II** 5 sets **LEVEL III** 7 sets **REST** up to 2 minutes

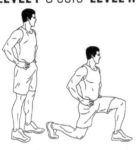

20 lunges

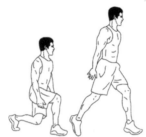

10 jumping lunges

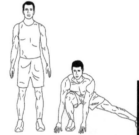

10 side lunges

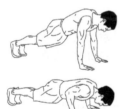

10 push-ups

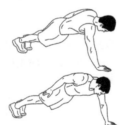

10 thigh taps

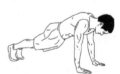

10-count plank

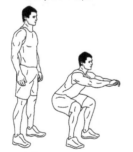

20 squats

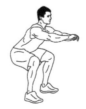

10-count squat hold

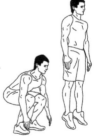

10 jump squats

58 Gravity Workout

To escape gravity you need dense muscles and strong bones and nothing gets muscles denser or bones stronger than a hyper-loaded floor workout.

Tip: There is little recovery time for each muscle group here so you need to make sure that your muscles get as much oxygen as possible by breathing in as deeply as possible at the recovery phase of each rep.

Gravity

DAREBEE WORKOUT © darebee.com

LEVEL I 3 sets **LEVEL II** 4 sets **LEVEL III** 5 sets **REST** 2 minutes

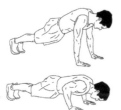

4 push-ups

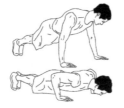

4 wide grip

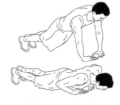

2 close grip

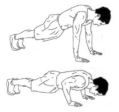

4 push-ups

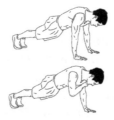

4 shoulder taps

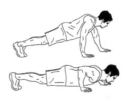

2 staggered

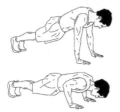

4 push-ups

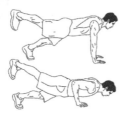

4 raised leg

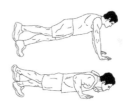

2 stacked feet

59 Guardian Workout

You know just by the name of the workout that it's going to be a little challenging. A guardian is never needed unless there is something to 'guard' which means it is worth fighting over for, which means that you'd better shape up if you want to play this role. The Guardian workout will test every aspect of your fitness.

Make it better: When performing side leg raises lean towards the leg you are raising, making your obliques work harder.

GUARDIAN

DAREBEE WORKOUT © darebee.com

LEVEL I 3 sets **LEVEL II** 5 sets **LEVEL III** 7 sets **REST** up to 2 minutes

STRENGTH

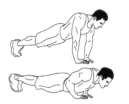

10 squats

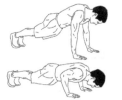

20 side leg raises

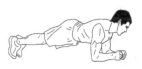

10 lunges

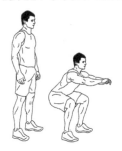

5 close grip push-ups

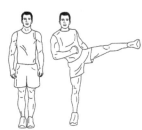

10 push-ups

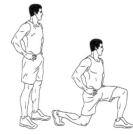

10-count elbow plank

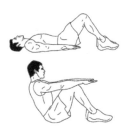

10 sit-ups

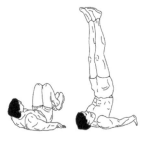

10 butt-ups

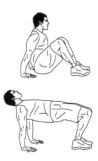

10 full bridges

60   Hercules Workout

Even a demigod needs to do something to maintain his strength. This is the workout for those who are readying themselves to join the ranks of the Olympian pantheon and have to perform a few labours beforehand.

HERCULES

DAREBEE WORKOUT © darebee.com

LEVEL I 3 sets **LEVEL II** 5 sets **LEVEL III** 7 sets **REST** up to 2 minutes

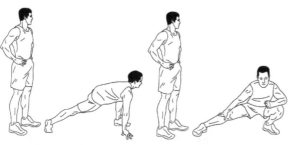

20combos lunge + deep side lunge

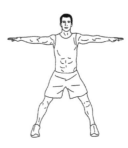

40-count star hold

STRENGTH

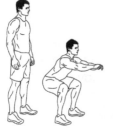

20combos squat + push-up

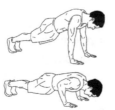

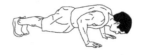

20-count push-up plank

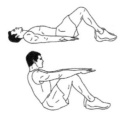

20combos sit-up + sitting twists

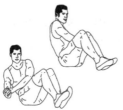

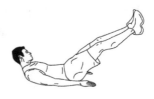

40-count raised leg hold

61 Homemade Back Workout

Your back muscles are important not just because you need something sturdy to rest upon when you get to bed at night but also because they power all sorts of subtle body movements, from the power of punches thrown from the hip to how well you perform at pull ups and how strong your overhead throw is. The Homemade Back workout targets all the major muscle groups of your back without forgetting some other, equally important parts of your body.

Make it harder: Balance on the balls of your feet for all standing exercises and challenge your core.

HOMEMADE BACK

DAREBEE WORKOUT
© darebee.com
LEVEL I 3 sets
LEVEL II 5 sets
LEVEL III 7 sets
REST up to 2 minutes

STRENGTH

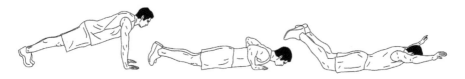

10 diver push-ups

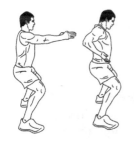

20 half squat rows

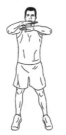
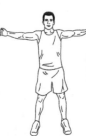

20 double chest expansions

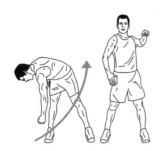

20 lawnmowers

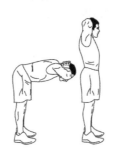

20 forward bends

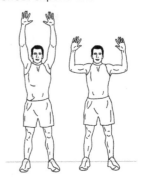

20 wall arm slides

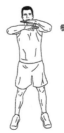

62 Huntsman Workout

Upper body strength requires a good strong core, pecs of steel and a strong lower back that connects the upper and lower parts of the trunk. The Huntsman workout takes you through a variety of push ups that require the coordination of the entire body, helping develop total body strength and greater overall power. Breathe in on the way down, exhale on the way up and remember to keep your body absolutely straight at all times.

Huntsman

DAREBEE WORKOUT © darebee.com
LEVEL I 2 reps LEVEL II 4 reps LEVEL III 6 reps each
LEVEL I 3 sets LEVEL II 5 sets LEVEL III 7 sets
REST up to 2 minutes

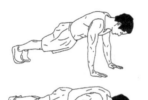

tricep push-ups

push-ups

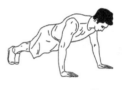
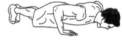

wide grip push-ups

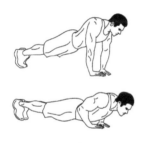

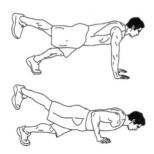

raised leg push-ups

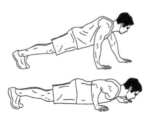

staggered push-ups

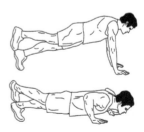

stacked push-ups

63 Leg Day Workout

Legs are what you need to use when you want to run (from zombies, werewolves and vampires, for example) and they're also kinda useful in everyday life because we still walk to get to places. This is a workout to help you make them strong and capable of performing at will.

Leg Day

DAREBEE WORKOUT © darebee.com

LEVEL I 3 sets **LEVEL II** 4 sets **LEVEL III** 5 sets **REST** up to 2 minutes

STRENGTH

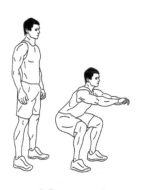

40 squats

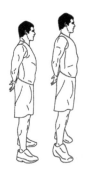

20 calf raises

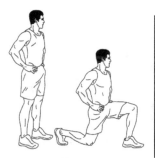

20 lunges

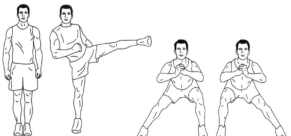

20 side leg raises

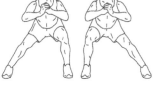

20 side-to-side lunges

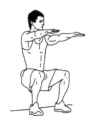

20-count wall-sit

64 Legs of Steel Workout

Your quads are the largest single muscle group in the body and your legs are needed to get you anywhere which is why the Legs of Steel workout will supercharge your quads and give you the kind of leg power that marks warriors from the rest.

Make it better: Perform everything on the balls of your feet.

legs of steel

DAREBEE WORKOUT © darebee.com

LEVEL I 3 sets **LEVEL II** 4 sets **LEVEL III** 5 sets **REST** up to 2 minutes

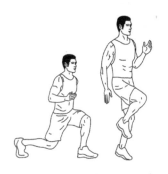

20 lunge steps-ups

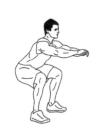

20sec squat hold

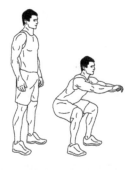

20 squats

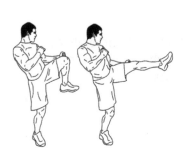

10 front kicks

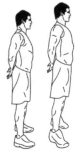

10 calf raises

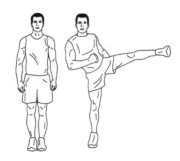

10 side leg raises

65 Odin Workout

Valhalla is a place where the gods don't just drink and revel but also train and fight. The Wrath of Odin workout is for those ready to prepare for that kind of 'revel' by punishing their body. Good for the soul and probably the closest you get to feeling like a Norse god.

Make it better: Perform punch combinations on the balls of your feet swiveling to bring your bodyweight behind each punch and further challenging your core, in the process.

THE WRATH OF
ODIN

DAREBEE WORKOUT © darebee.com

LEVEL I 3 sets **LEVEL II** 5 sets **LEVEL III** 7 sets **REST** up to 2 minutes

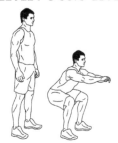
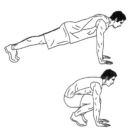
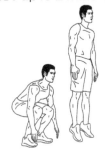

20combos squat   +   plank jump-in   +   jump squat

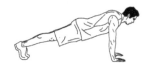
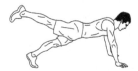
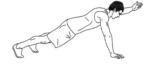

10-count each plank   +   raised leg plank   +   raised arm plank

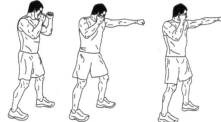
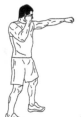
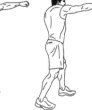
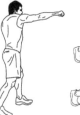
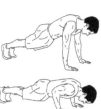

20combos   jab   +   jab   +   cross   +   push-up

66 Paladin Workout

Total body strength revolves around a core and the Paladin workout works the core in different ways bringing relevant muscle groups into play and helping you increase trunk stability and posture holding.

Make it better: Make sure you have pulled in your lower abs tight against your spine to align the ab wall muscles better.

PALADIN

DAREBEE WORKOUT © darebee.com
LEVEL I 2 reps **LEVEL II** 4 reps **LEVEL III** 6 reps each
LEVEL I 3 sets **LEVEL II** 4 sets **LEVEL III** 5 sets **REST** up to 2 minutes

STRENGTH

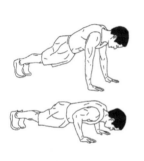

push-ups

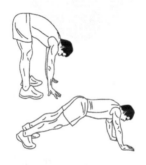

plank walk-outs

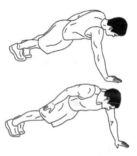

thigh taps

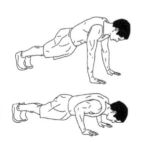

push-ups

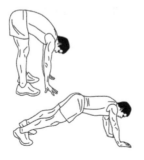

plank walk-outs

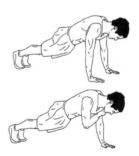

shoulder taps

67 Plan B Workout

A Plan B workout is there for when there is no plan A. This is a 'gentle' workout. It won't push you to the limits, you won't be reduced to swearing under your breath and there won't even be much muscle soreness the day after, but it will still give you a decent workout which is definitely better than none.

Make it better: Make sure your squats are a perfect 90 degree angle.

PLAN B

DAREBEE WORKOUT © darebee.com
LEVEL I 3 sets **LEVEL II** 5 sets **LEVEL III** 7 sets **REST** up to 2 minutes

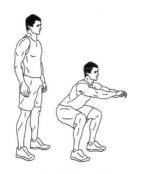

20 squats

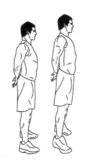

20 calf raises

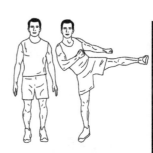

20 side leg raises

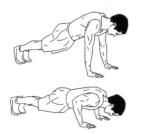

10 push-ups

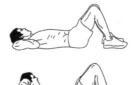

10 crunches

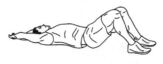
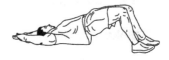

10 bridges

68 Power Flow Workout

Exercise is deceptive. Take two things that can be done easily, put them one after the other, demand that the body flows from one to the other and suddenly you begin to wonder what kind of hell you've wondered into. This is why ballet, gymnastics or martial arts are so difficult. Somehow the "flow" requires more attention, more balance and greater concentration than any simple start/stop exercise. PowerFlow is a workout that will make you sweat and then some. It will also make you fitter, stronger, faster and more durable than you ever imagined. And it will do it quickly.

Make it harder: Do it faster.

Power Flow

DAREBEE WORKOUT © darebee.com
repeat the sequence 20 times = 1 set
LEVEL I 3 sets   **LEVEL II** 4 sets   **LEVEL III** 5 sets
up to 2 minutes rest between sets

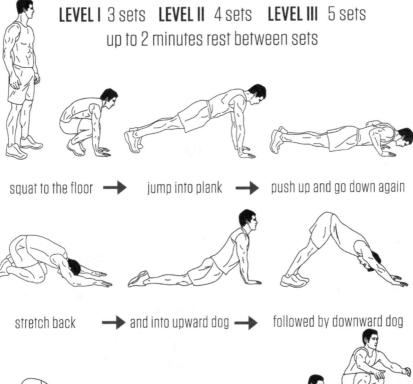

squat to the floor ➡ jump into plank ➡ push up and go down again

stretch back ➡ and into upward dog ➡ followed by downward dog

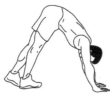
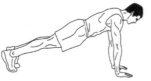
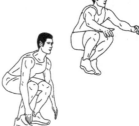
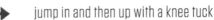

slowly walk back into a plank ➡ jump in and then up with a knee tuck

.69 Power Mode Workout

Strength is the ability of the muscles to perform work at a high intensity consistently and it is build, over time, by making muscle groups work under load on the entire muscle fiber. This is a workout that is performed deliberately and with focus. Attention is paid to technique so that form is maintained. You won't get out of breath but you will work up a sweat.

Make it better: Slow everything down a little. By removing the ballistic movement element from the workout you force your muscles to use all their strength.

POWER MODE

DAREBEE WORKOUT © darebee.com

LEVEL I 3 sets **LEVEL II** 5 sets **LEVEL III** 7 sets **REST** up to 2 minutes

STRENGTH

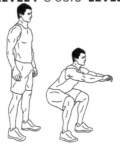

20 squats

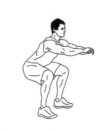

20-count squat hold

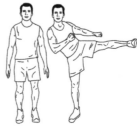

20 side leg raises

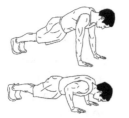

10 push-ups

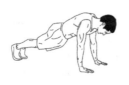

10-count plank

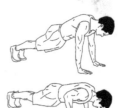

10 push-ups

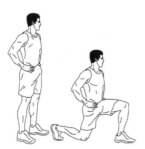

20 lunges

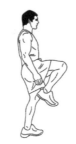

20-count balance hold

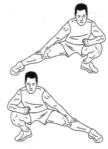

20 side lunges

70 Primal Workout

Go native and let your body move with an atavistic sense of power and grace with our Primal workout. Whether you hop like a Kangaroo, or sting like a Scorpion there is an element of fun to the challenge that makes the workout addictive. So unleash the animals inside yourself. All of them. And feel the power flowing through your muscles.

Make it better: Add some animal noises as you perform the exercises, you'll be surprised at the difference it actually makes to your performance (once you get over your shyness, that is).

PRIMAL

DAREBEE WORKOUT © darebee.com

LEVEL I 3 sets **LEVEL II** 5 sets **LEVEL III** 7 sets **REST** up to 2 minutes

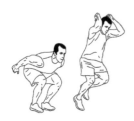

20 hops

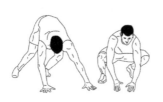

20 side-to-side hops

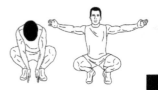

20 ape reaches

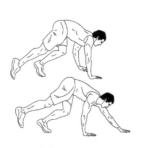

10 bear crawl

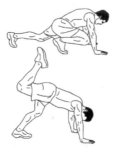

10 scorpion reaches

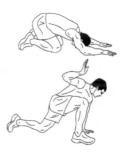

10 front steps

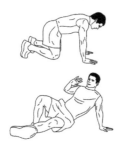

10 sit-outs

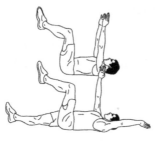

10 dead bugs

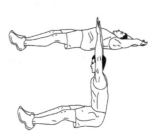

10 L-situps

71 Push, Squat, Repeat Workout

Sometimes what you want is to be able to simply do something simple. No overthinking the part, no role-play in your head. Nothing that will constantly challenge your coordination and force you to be mindful of your body every single moment of the workout. This is where this "Wash, Rinse and Repeat" cycle is perfect. You can set it up and let your body do its thing while your mind takes a figurative break for a while. So, choose your level and get ready to rock it.

Make it harder: Train like a boxing legend. Cut down your recovery time between sets to just 30 seconds.

DAREBEE WORKOUT
© darebee.com
LEVEL I 3 sets
LEVEL II 5 sets
LEVEL III 7 sets
REST up to 2 minutes

PUSH SQUAT REPEAT

STRENGTH

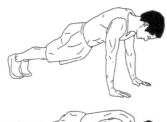
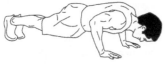
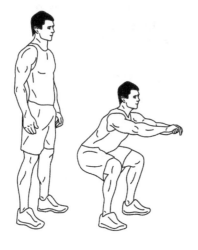

4 reps	push-ups
4 reps	squats
10 reps	push-ups
10 reps	squats
4 reps	push-ups
4 reps	squats
10 reps	push-ups
10 reps	squats
	rest

72   Reaper Workout

A strong core affects everything. Your balance is better. The supporting muscle groups work faster. You feel stronger. You are more in control of your body. Everything you do feels more powerful. The Reaper workout works your core and attendant abdominal muscle groups for a lean, strong look.

Make it better: Keep your body absolutely straight in every plank and every push up by lightly tensing your lower abs.

REAPER

DAREBEE WORKOUT © darebee.com

LEVEL I 3 sets **LEVEL II** 4 sets **LEVEL III** 5 sets **REST** up to 2 minutes

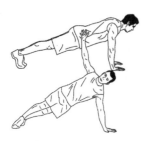 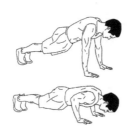 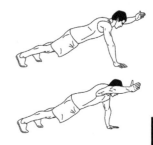

10combos plank rotations + push-up + plank arm raises

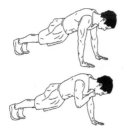 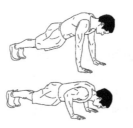 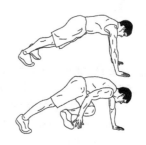

10combos shoulder taps + push-up + climber taps

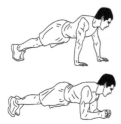 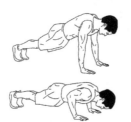 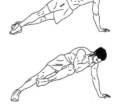

10combos up & down plank + push-up + side plank crunches

73 Reclaimer Workout

The Reclaimer workout helps you get back control of your core, abs and obliques and the supporting muscle groups that are called upon every time you need to push the envelope of your performance. You should do this after a light warm-up for maximum results.

Make it better: Pick up speed without sacrificing form, try and perform each set a little bit faster.

Reclaimer

DAREBEE WORKOUT © darebee.com

LEVEL I 3 sets **LEVEL II** 5 sets **LEVEL III** 7 sets **REST** up to 2 minutes

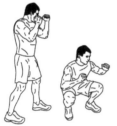

10 combos squat + push-ups

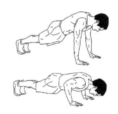

10 slow push-ups

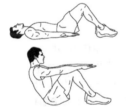

10 sit-ups

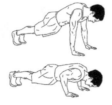

10 sitting twists

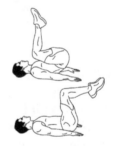

10 reverse crunches

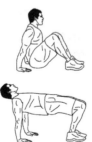

10 full bridges

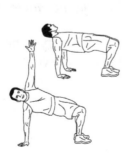

10 full bridges with reach

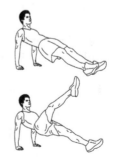

10 reverse plank leg raises

74 Savage Workout

When it's time to get savage on your upper body, make your shoulders scream for mercy a little and push your lungs to work that extra bit faster the Savage work out goes a little medieval on your arms. Moving from hyperloading to ballistic movements and demanding both concentric and eccentric muscle fiber movements it will make your arms beg for mercy. Be deaf to their pleas and just get through the workout.

Make it harder: Pick up the speed, try to beat your own time in completing each set and challenge your aerobic performance.

SAVAGE

DAREBEE WORKOUT © darebee.com

LEVEL I 3 sets **LEVEL II** 4 sets **LEVEL III** 5 sets **REST** up to 2 minutes

STRENGTH

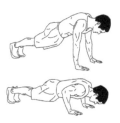

5 push-ups

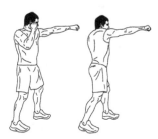

10 punches

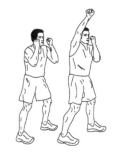

10 overhead punches

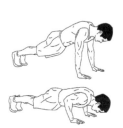

5 push-ups

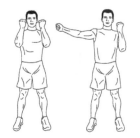

10 side-to-side backfists

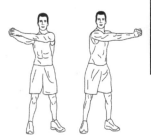

10 side-to-side chops

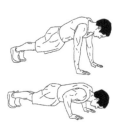

5 push-ups

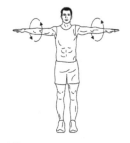

10 raised arm circles

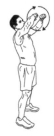

10 speed bag punches

75 Sculptor Workout

Sculpt your body, up your speed and push your aerobic performance to new heights with the Sculptor workout. This combines it all plus the slow exercises at the end of each combo force you to use your muscles fully.

Make it better: Go super slow on each slow exercise.

SCULPTOR

DAREBEE WORKOUT © darebee.com

LEVEL I 3 sets **LEVEL II** 5 sets **LEVEL III** 7 sets **REST** up to 2 minutes

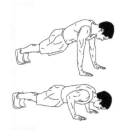 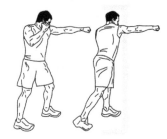 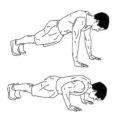

4combos: **2** push-up + **10** jab + cross   **10** slow push-ups

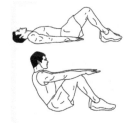 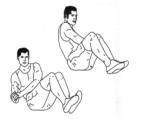 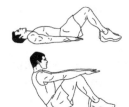

4combos: **2** sit-ups + **10** sitting twists   **10** slow sit-ups

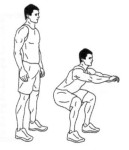 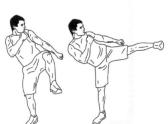 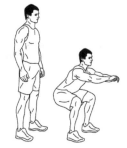

4combos: **2** squats + **10** side kicks   **10** slow squats

76 Spartan Workout

Spartans took pain and made it their friend. The Spartan workout exercises some major muscle groups to give you the total warrior feeling when you move.

Tip: When doing push-ups and lunges make sure your back is as straight as possible. This ensures that pressure is applied to the muscles more evenly and avoids any possible, lower back injury.

SPARTAN

DAREBEE WORKOUT © darebee.com

LEVEL I 3 sets **LEVEL II** 5 sets **LEVEL III** 7 sets **REST** up to 2 minutes

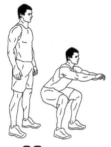

20 squats

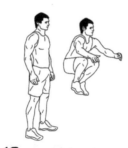

10 jump knee tucks

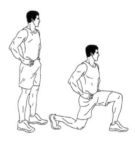

20 lunges

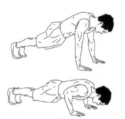

10 push-ups

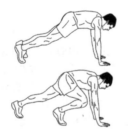

10 slow climbers

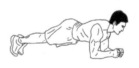

10-count elbow plank

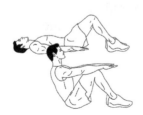

10 sit-ups

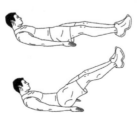

10 leg raises

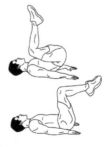

10 reverse crunches

77 Super Soldier Workout

There are few workouts that will give you a strength challenge in as short a time as the Super Soldier one. In a gradual way it loads all the major muscle groups, making them work isometrically or eccentrically, bringing up the body's temperature and activating the cardiovascular system but without challenging aerobic performance.

Make it harder: Slow the push ups down a little so you do them deep and slow. Slow the knee-to-elbow crunches a little so that you are using your internal and external obliques to control the movement.

SUPER SOLDIER

DAREBEE WORKOUT © darebee.com

LEVEL I 3 sets **LEVEL II** 5 sets **LEVEL III** 7 sets **REST** up to 2 minutes

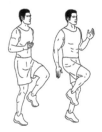

20 squats

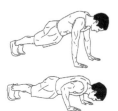

10 push-ups

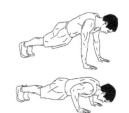

10-count push-up

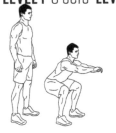

3 combos: **20** high knees + **1** jump knee tuck

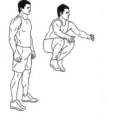

10 army crawl

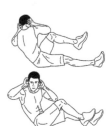

10 knee-to-elbow crunches

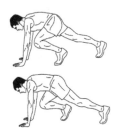

20 climbers

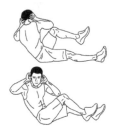

10 knee-to-elbow crunches

78   Titan Workout

Impossible acts require exceptional focus. When you are a warrior of the Light, your Destiny lies in surviving against dire odds by levelling up fast. The Titan workout will get you there faster and the faster you do it, the better you'll be ... Guardian.

Make it better: When performing high crunches keep your chin on your chest at all times, working your neck muscles and activating your upper abdominals.

TITAN

DAREBEE WORKOUT © darebee.com

LEVEL I 3 sets **LEVEL II** 5 sets **LEVEL III** 7 sets **REST** up to 2 minutes

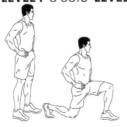

20 lunges

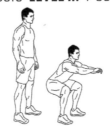

20 squats

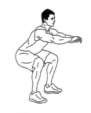

20-count squat hold

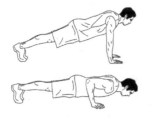

10 push-ups

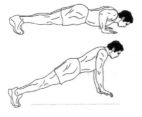

4 power push-ups

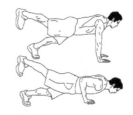

4 raised leg push-ups

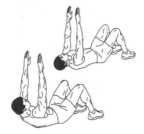

10 high crunches

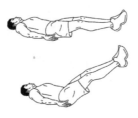

10 leg raises

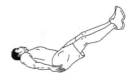

10-count raised leg hold

79 Viking Workout

It takes a special kind of warrior to brave the open seas on a shallow-keel boat and go raiding for riches. Physical presence is a given. A sense of raw power comes with the territory. And giving up is simply not an option. How you get to be like that is very much part of the physical workout you subject yourself to. Your body is always a work-in-progress. It responds to the physical demands made upon it. The Vikings were physically formidable because they lived in an environment that naturally favoured only the survival of the fittest. That ensured that even the weakest amongst them was more than capable of taking care of himself. This is one workout which you know you need to add to your training even if you don't go raiding along the English coastline every summer.

VIKING

DAREBEE WORKOUT © darebee.com

LEVEL I 3 sets **LEVEL II** 5 sets **LEVEL III** 7 sets **REST** up to 2 minutes

STRENGTH

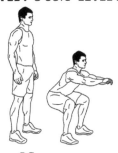

20 squats

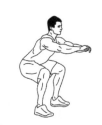

20-count squat hold

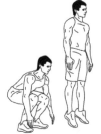

4 jump squats

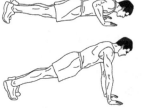

20 push-ups

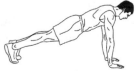

20-count plank hold

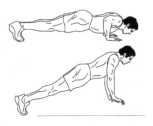

4 power push-ups

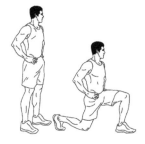

20 lunges

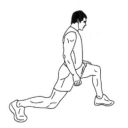

20-count deep lunge hold

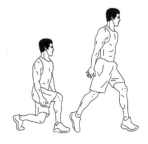

4 jumping lunges

80 Anchor'd Workout

Active stretching demands you assume a position and then hold it using nothing but the strength of the agonist muscles. The results of active stretching are not just elongated muscles but also enhanced muscle growth, stronger tendons and a greater range of motion in the main muscle groups afterwards The Anchor'd active stretching workout takes you through some of the key positions that affect the body's main muscle groups. You will feel the difference afterwards.

Make it harder: Take no rest between sets.

ANCHOR'D

ACTIVE STRETCHING © darebee.com

60 seconds each - 30 seconds each leg

3 sets | up to 2 minutes rest between sets

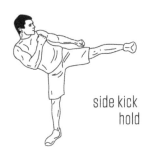

side kick
hold

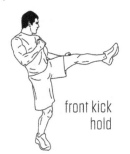

front kick
hold

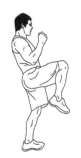

raised
knee
hold

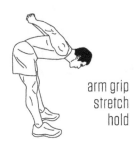

arm grip
stretch
hold

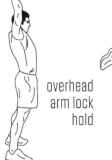

overhead
arm lock
hold

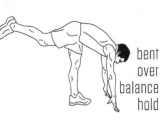

bent
over
balance
hold

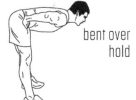

bent over
hold

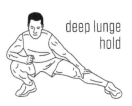

deep lunge
hold

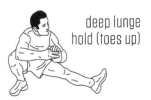

deep lunge
hold (toes up)

FLEXIBILITY

81 Balance & Coordination

A good balance is the result of a strong core, stable tendons and powerful support muscle groups. Balance exercises help develop the muscle groups and tendons needed for developing muscular control, great physical prowess and the kind of body strength that marks true athletes.

Make it harder: Try to form a perfect "T" shape with your body when performing the balance stand. It's way harder than you think and sweat will flow.

BALANCE &
COORDINATION

DAREBEE WORKOUT © darebee.com

LEVEL I 3 sets **LEVEL II** 5 sets **LEVEL III** 7 sets **REST** up to 2 minutes
Repeat the sequence going from one move to the next quickly
10 times in total (5 each side) = 1 set

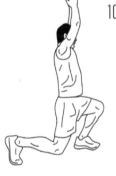

lunge

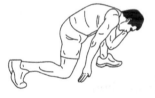

deep lunge elbow bent

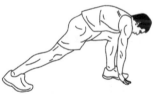

deep lunge

FLEXIBILITY

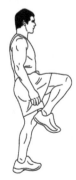

knee raise

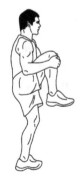

knee raise press

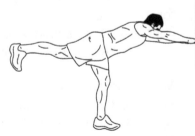

balance stand

82   Bowman Workout

PNF stretching which is also known as proprioceptive neuromuscular facilitation stretching, is a set of stretching techniques that can increase both active and passive range of motion and provide real gains in flexibility in a really short time. Treating your body almost like a bow you pull to your maximum range while resisting, hold it long enough (usually 15 seconds) for the muscles and tendons to tire and the appropriate muscle fiber relaxation response to kick in and then you apply pressure again, stretching the muscles even more.

Make it better: PNF is all about pushing the limites every time. The pull/resist-hold-relax-pull again routine allows your muscles to stretch beyond their normal range, quickly and increases plasticity.

BOWMAN

PNF STRETCHIN © darebee.com
60 seconds each - 30 seconds each side / leg
3 sets | up to 2 minutes rest between sets
Pull for 15 seconds while resisting. Relax and pull again.

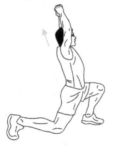

leg to chest stretch   legs back stretch   legs apart stretch

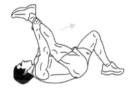
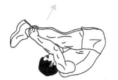
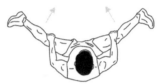

heel hold stretch   lunge back stretch   lunge tilt stretch

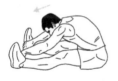
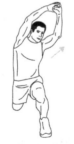

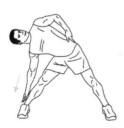
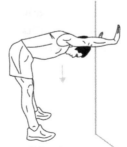
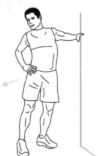

side stretches   wall bent over   wall body tilt

FLEXIBILITY

83   Far Point Workout

Passive stretching is an ideal form of stretching to perform with a partner. It requires the body to remain completely passive while an outside force is exerted upon it (by a partner). When used without a partner bodyweight and the force of gravity are allowed to do their thing. Passive stretching is also called relaxed stretching, for that reason. To make it work for you, extend to a position that is at the very edge of your comfort zone and hold it, allowing gravity and your bodyweight to do the rest. There is no 'bounce' of any kind with passive stretching, nor is there any push/pull motion.

FAR POINT

PASSIVE STRETCHING © darebee.com

60 seconds each - 30 seconds each side / leg

3 sets | up to 2 minutes rest between sets

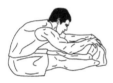

hamstring stretch

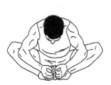

groin stretch

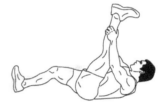

leg to chest stretch

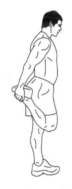

quad stretch

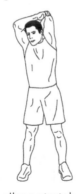

elbow stretch

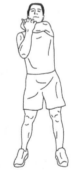

cross neck elbow stretch

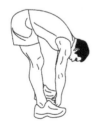

gravity toe touches

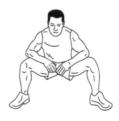

sumo squat hold

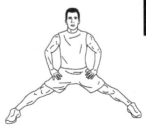

side splits

FLEXIBILITY

84 Inner Warrior Workout

Unleash your inner warrior by activating all your muscles in a series of exercises that challenge strength, balance and include stretching. The Inner Warrior workout uses Yoga poses in a flowing sequence that will leave you feeling totally energized, your body fully awakened and your muscles flowing smoothly. All you need is a little space, a little time and some inner peace of mind to allow you to concentrate on what your body is doing. The Inner Warrior workout can be coupled with power breathing to help your abdominals get stronger faster and aid your aerobic development.

INNER
WARRIOR

DAREBEE WORKOUT © darebee.com
LEVEL I 3 sets **LEVEL II** 5 sets **LEVEL III** 7 sets
REST up to 2 minutes

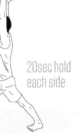
20sec hold
each side

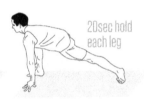
20sec hold
each side

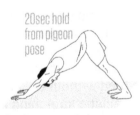
20sec hold
each leg

1. warrior I   2. warrior II   3. lunge

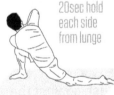
20sec hold
each side
from lunge

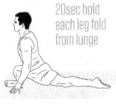
20sec hold
each leg fold
from lunge

20sec hold
from pigeon
pose

4. lunge with twist   5. pigeon pose   6. downward dog

20sec hold
from downward dog

20sec hold
from bow pose

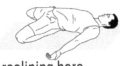
20sec hold
from child pose

7. bow pose   8. child pose   9. reclining hero

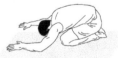

FLEXIBILITY

85 Liber8 Workout

Ballistic stretching is a form of stretching that uses bounce and muscle explosion to force a stretch through a range of movement or a fixed position. Because ballistic stretching pushes the body beyond its comfort zone it should never be tried without an adequate warm-up. The Liber8 workout is a ballistic stretching routine that allows you to push against the current boundaries of your flexibility and begin to make some gains. Liberate your body.

Make it harder: Don't rest between sets and increase the temperature of your muscles and their ability to stretch.

Liber8

BALLISTIC STRETCHING BY DAREBEE © darebee.com

40 reps each | 3 sets | up to 2 minutes rest between sets

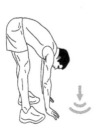

bent over reach

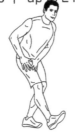

hamstring stretch

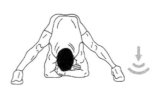

body fold floor reach

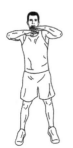

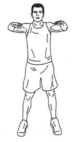

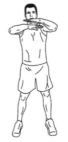

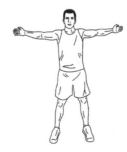

double chest expansions

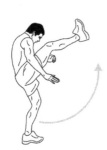

high front kick

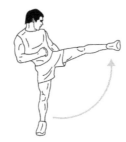

high side leg raises

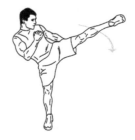

high turning kicks

86   Origami Workout

Origami is about precision and this workout helps you develop precision in your movements by training the very muscle groups you need to give you better control of your body.

Tip: When performing the airplane balance, experiment having your standing leg with the knee bent and the knee straight. The latter challenges core balance a lot more and makes you work a lot harder.

origami

DAREBEE WORKOUT © darebee.com

3 sets | up to 2 minutes rest between sets
20 seconds each side / no rest between exercises

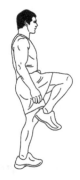

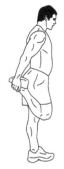

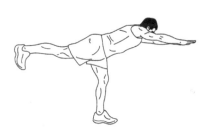

40sec raised knee   **40sec** one leg stand   **40sec** airplane balance

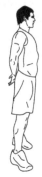

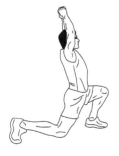

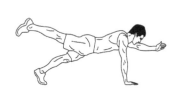

20sec calf raise hold   **40sec** lunge balance   **40sec** alt arm/leg plank

FLEXIBILITY

87   Steakout Workout

Combat moves in workouts aim to let you gain control over your body so that it truly becomes an instrument of your will. The Stakeout Workout takes you through a series of moves that will challenge your balance, flexibility and ballistic body movement. Combine it with executing most of these moves balancing on the balls of your feet and you have an instant challenge to your deep core abdominal muscles. Add speed and you up the aerobic element to it all.

steakout

ACTIVE STRETCHING © darebee.com
20 seconds each | 2 sets , one for each side
no rest between sets

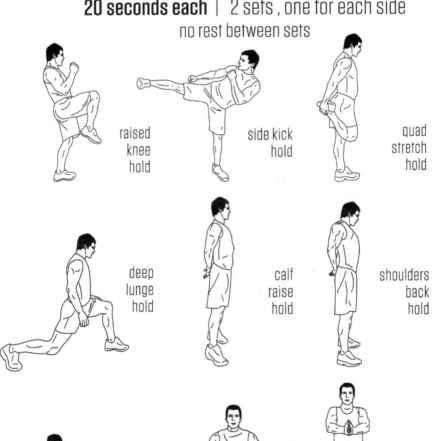

raised
knee
hold

side kick
hold

quad
stretch
hold

deep
lunge
hold

calf
raise
hold

shoulders
back
hold

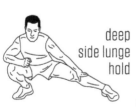

deep
side lunge
hold

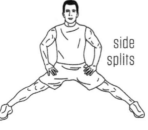

side
splits

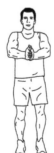

chest
squeeze

88 Express Workout

This is the workout for when you want something fast, are pressed for time but don't want to skimp on quality. Up the intensity just a little on each rep and you can both have your cake and eat it.

EXPRESS
WORKOUT

BY DAREBEE © darebee.com

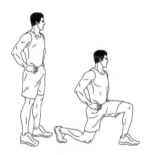

20 lunges

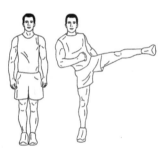

20 side leg raises

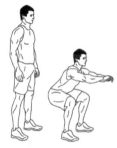

20 squats

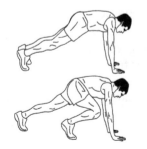

20 slow climber

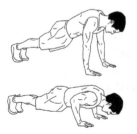

20 push-ups

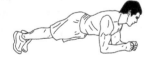

20sec elbow plank

MICRO

89   Coffee Break Workout

A coffee break is always great, especially if your day starts
with one, which then doesn't quite make it a break but there is
certainly coffee involved. Add some movement, throw in a little
need for balance and you've got yourself the kind of workout
Kung Fu legends are made of. Fill your cup almost to the brim
and you're beginning to get into the Jedi zone. The Coffee Break
workout may not look that challenging at first glance but try it
out with a cup that's filled almost to the brim and you will find it
takes incredible and muscle control to prevent it from spilling.
Exactly the kind of balance and muscle control that allow you to
move with the sureness of a panther and the speed of a snake.
Now go get that cup of coffee.

Coffee BREAK

DAREBEE WORKOUT © darebee.com
3 sets | up to 2 minutes rest between sets

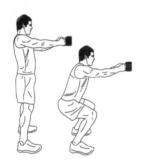

10 squats

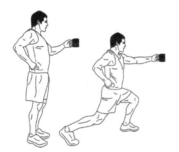

10 lunges

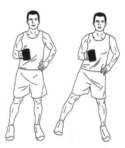

10 side leg swings

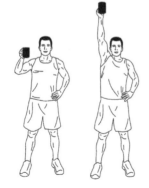

20 mug raises

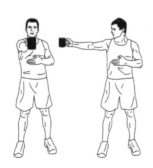

20 arm rotations

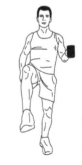

20-count hold

MICRO

90   Gamer Workout

Whether on-screen or off it a Gamer needs to have some sound core stability and strength and the ability to control his body to the max. This workout is a pretty good place to start for those qualities.

Tip: For lunges and squats to have their best result you need to push off with your legs in a smooth, fluid motion, exhaling as you do.

GAMER

DAREBEE WORKOUT © darebee.com
every respawn, construction or cinematic trailer

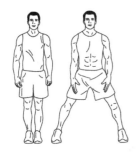

20 half jacks

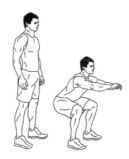

10 squats

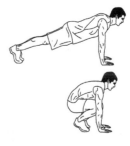

10 plank jump-ins

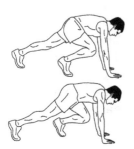

20 climbers

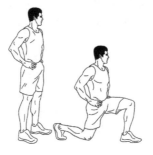

10 lunges

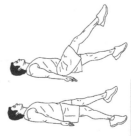

10 flutter kicks

MICRO

91 Hand Workout

Our hands are our greatest weapon. The human hand has enabled us to build civilizations, fight wars, play instruments and control machines. Without the hand even gaming becomes next to impossible. The human hand has 27 bones, not including the sesamoid bone, the number of which varies between people, 14 of which are the phalanges (proximal, intermediate and distal) of the fingers. The metacarpals are the bones that connect the fingers and the wrist. Each human hand has five metacarpals and 8 carpal bones. The Talk to the Hand workout helps you work them all, plus it has the added bonus of testing the power of the forearm muscles, increasing the strength of your grip and improving the overall dexterity of your hands.

TALK TO THE
HAND

DAREBEE
WORKOUT
© darebee.com
3 sets | 2 minutes rest

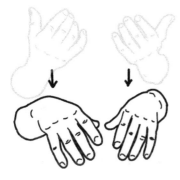

1. rapid shaking

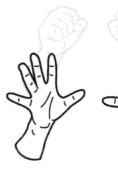

2. open and close fists

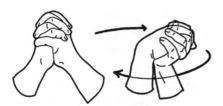

3. rotations

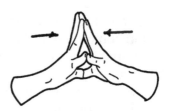

4. finger press

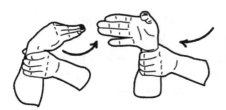

5. side flickers

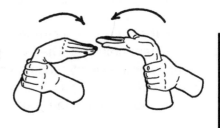

6. up and down wrist flips

MICRO

92 Movie Night Workout

You know that feeling when all you want to do is sit at home watching something on TV? The world outside has ceased to exist but that doesn't mean that your drive for fitness needs to go bye-bye. Quite the opposite in fact. Here's a chance to turn that sofa into your playground making the night-in movie your fitness aid. If you want to have your cake and eat it, this is the perfect way to start. So indulge, watch that film and chill at home and don't forget to make your reps count.

Make it better: You're sitting down so there is not a lot of movement going on when you punch. Take your punches to an entirely new level by tensing your biceps and clenching your fists tightly as you punch. This will increase the resistance load on the muscles making your arms work extra hard.

movie night

DAREBEE WORKOUT © darebee.com

Repeat 3 times | up to 2 minutes rest between sets
or every 20 minutes during a movie

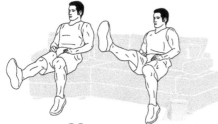

20 leg swings

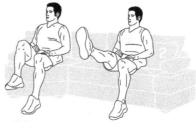

20 front snap kicks

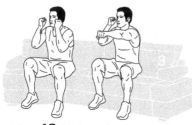

40 punches

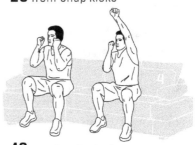

40 overhead punches

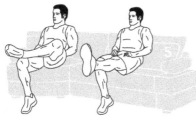

20 knee taps

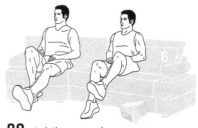

20 air bike crunches

MICRO

93   Office Workout

Just because you're at the office does not mean you can't workout. This is the kind of exercise routine that can be carried out anywhere you have a little space and some privacy.

Tip: None of this need be done fast. You are, after all, at the office. But do them in a focused way and they help you work out every single muscle group of your body.

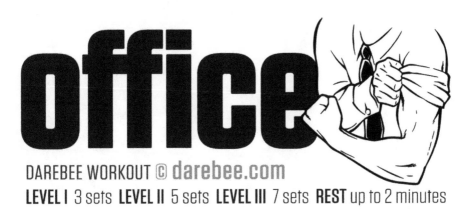

office

DAREBEE WORKOUT © **darebee.com**

LEVEL I 3 sets **LEVEL II** 5 sets **LEVEL III** 7 sets **REST** up to 2 minutes

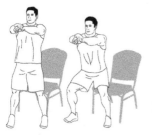

20 chair squats

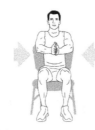

20 chest squeezes

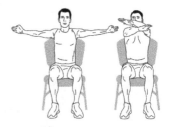

40 criss-cross arms

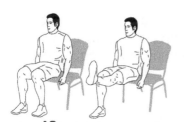

40 leg extensions

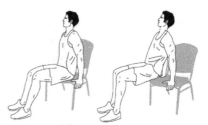

10 chair body lifts

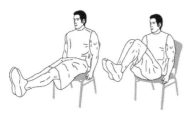

10 knee pull-ins

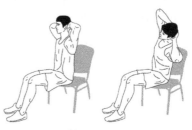

20 oblique bends

MICRO

94 Sofa Abs Workout

At the end of a busy day, all you want is the chance to put work out of your mind, land on the sofa, turn the telly on and ... work your abs. The sofa's your gym. Your body is your equipment. This is the Sofa Abs workout. If you're on the sofa, it's time to work your abs.

Make it harder: You shouldn't. It's a sofa workout, after all but if you happen to have a pair of ankle weights lying around, now's the time to strap them on.

sofa abs

DAREBEE WORKOUT © darebee.com

LEVEL I 3 sets **LEVEL II** 4 sets **LEVEL III** 5 sets **REST** up to 2 minutes

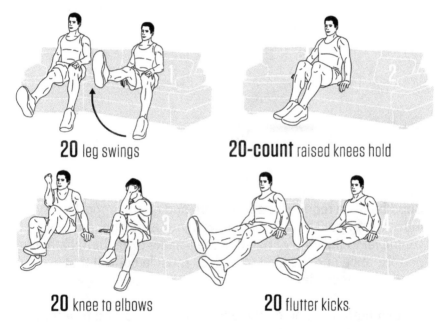

20 leg swings

20-count raised knees hold

20 knee to elbows

20 flutter kicks

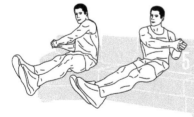

10 raised legs twists

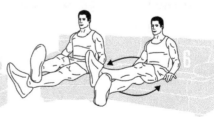

10 scissors

MICRO

95   Star Master Workout

Good balance requires a strong core and great supporting muscle groups. The Star Master workout is designed to help you develop the kind of balance that marks exceptional athletic performance and the kind of badass muscle control that warrior-types achieve.

Make it better: Stand on the ball of your supporting foot for an even greater challenge to your balance.

Star Master

DAREBEE WORKOUT © darebee.com

Instructions: balance on one leg and tap with the other.

3 minutes right leg clockwise
3 minutes left leg counterclockwise
6 minutes in total

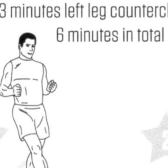

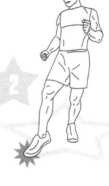

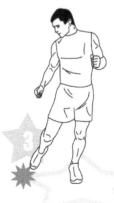

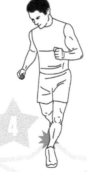

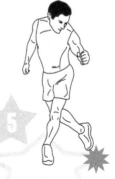

MICRO

96   Wake Up! Workout

Start the day with a bang with a workout that'll get your pulse going and get your energy levels up.

Tip: This is a fast, light workout designed to help you get your body going in the morning. Take deep, even breaths, throughout to help you start the day with an inner glow.

WAKE UP!
& MAKE IT HAPPEN

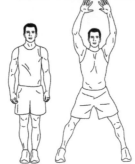

20 jumping jacks

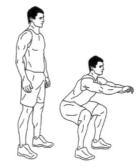

20 squats

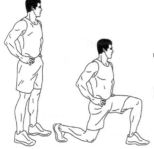

10 lunges

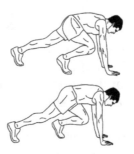

10 climbers

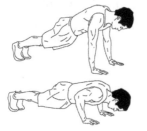

10 push-ups

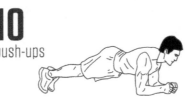

20sec elbow plank

MICRO

97 Knee Workout

Knees take a pounding even before an arrow happens to find them. Because the knee is a hinge type synovial joint it presents a level of complexity not seen in other joints. Conditioning of the surrounding muscles is crucial in achieving joint stability and preventing injury. If you have been unlucky enough to have been injured here, the exercises will help add to the speed of rehabilitation of the knee joint (as long as you are not at one of the stages of injury that require operational intervention). The exercises here are designed to help maintain the range of motion a healthy knee joint is capable of. They can also work as preventative measures, taken to avoid sustaining knee injuries.

KNEE

REHAB WORKOUT
© darebee.com
LEVEL I 3 sets
LEVEL II 5 sets
LEVEL III 7 sets
REST up to 2 minutes

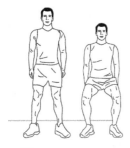

10 wall half squats

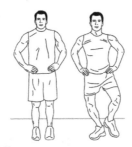

10 wide single leg squats

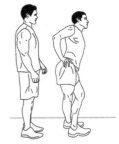

30sec cross leg side tilts

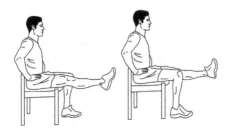

10 leg raises

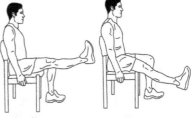

20 raised leg swings

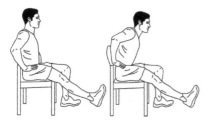

30sec hamstring stretch

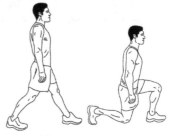

10 split squats

REHAB

98 Lower Back Workout

The lower back is a weak link in our anatomy not because we are not supposed to stand up on our hind legs, but because we spend so much of our lives sitting down. The Lower Back workout, developed in cooperation with NHS specialists (British National Health Service) is designed to help you activate your back, work it gently so that the muscles align and any pain you may be experiencing, slowly goes away. Practice it any time you feel your lower back acting up and make it part of your training regime as a preventative measure.

LOWER BACK

REHAB WORKOUT
© darebee.com
3 sets | 2 minutes rest

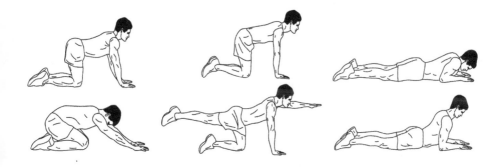

10 bottom to heels stretch   **10** opposite arm / leg raises   **10** back extensions

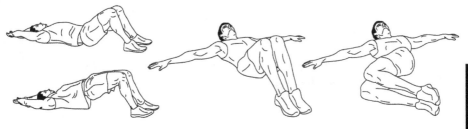

10 bridges   **10** knee rolls

REHAB

99   Man Down Workout

Change your perspective on the world, and training, with the "Man Down" workout. Stretch, arch and reach, turning your body into a performing machine as you put it through its paces. When you do not have to fight gravity too much you begin to rediscover fresh control over your muscles. This is your recovery workout, performed each time you don't quite feel like working out.

Make it harder: Bring your chin to your chest when performing bridges making your upper abs tense up and working your lower back and glutes harder against them.

man down

DAREBEE WORKOUT © darebee.com
3 sets | up to 2 minutes rest between sets

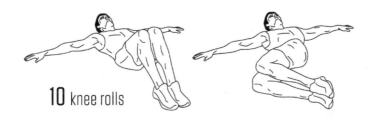

10 knee rolls

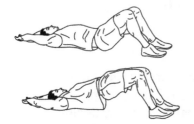

10 bridges

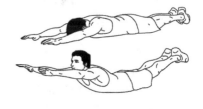

10 x 10sec stretch & hold

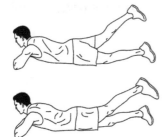

10 reverse flutter kicks

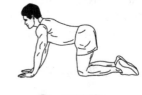
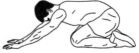

10 x 5sec stretch & hold

MICRO

100   Neck Workout

Neck pain is one of the most common complaints of our digitally-enhanced society. Time spent in front of screens or looking at our devices, insufficient focus on neck muscles during our workouts and too little time to spend on this muscle group in general contribute to frequent complaints. The Neck Pain and Tension Relief workout remedies all those problems. It can be performed as a warm-up, before exercise or as a total stress reliever at the end of the day.

Make it harder: In this case this is as hard as it should be.

NECK

DAREBEE WORKOUT
© darebee.com
3 sets | 2 minutes rest

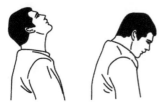

10 back and forth tilts

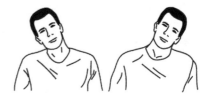

10 side-to-side tilts

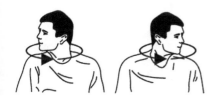

10 neck rotations

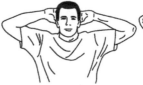

10-count press

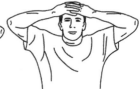

10-count press

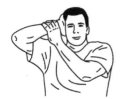
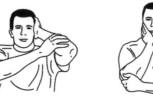

10-count alternating side press

10-count alternating chin press

Fitness is a journey, not a destination.
Darebee, Project

CPSIA information can be obtained
at www.ICGtesting.com
Printed in the USA
BVHW062236090920
588458BV00011B/402